CHANGE IS COMING

A Holistic Guide to Navigating
Menopause with Confidence

LYNETTE SADLER

Conscious Dreams
PUBLISHING

Change is Coming

Copyright © 2025: Lynette Sadler

This book does not provide medical or legal advice. It is for information purposes only. The medical and/or nutritional information in this book is not intended to be a substitute for professional medical advice, diagnosis, or treatment. Always seek the advice of your Doctor or other qualified health provider with any questions you may have regarding a medical condition.

First Printed in United Kingdom 2018

Published by Conscious Dreams Publishing
www.consciousdreamspublishing.com

Book Consultant Daniella Blechner

Edited by Elise Abram

Typeset by Oksana Kosovan

ISBN: 978-1-912551-46-0

Dedicated to you, the reader,
who wishes to reclaim your health and help your family
and friends to do the same.

Acknowledgements

My gratitude to my family, friends and colleagues who encouraged me on this journey. I also extend my deepest gratitude to my sons, Marlon and Leon Sadler, who motivated and inspired me to write this book. Your self-belief knows no bounds.

A special thanks to the Conscious Dreams Publishing team who assisted me in many areas of this project. Daniella Blechner, Book Journey Mentor, Elise Abram, editor, Oksana Kosovan, typesetter and cover designer, Emily's World of Design. I am equally grateful to Shahenara Begum for her assistance with the illustrations.

Contents

Introduction

To say I was unprepared for The Change is an understatement. Beset with health woes spanning nearly 16 years, I decided it was crucial for me to take control of my health and take the necessary steps to improve my wellbeing. Now, in my middle years, the nagging thoughts at the back of my mind are at the forefront, prodding me to make changes. The plight of those close to me who lost their lives due to illnesses or who were experiencing ailments such as hypertension, cancer, fibroids, diabetes and allergies that most health professionals would say were avoidable screamed at me to sit up and pay attention. However, it was not until my hormones started to 'malfunction' that I embarked on my quest to find out how I could get back on track.

Having read numerous articles on health for midlife women, I discovered a common theme: food. I learnt that what we eat is an issue and that we have to take control of it as we face The Change.

Questions popped up in my mind, one after another, like flickering lights: Was my diet having an impact on my health? Was my so-called healthy diet not as healthy as I once thought? More research led me to the conclusion that my diet was likely the root of the symptoms that had plagued me for years and equally affected the function of my hormones. What I discovered about food will not only surprise you, but it will make you more cautious about what you put on your plate, and all the more so as you enter The Change.

Hormone replacement therapy (HRT) was an option I wanted to avoid primarily because of the side effects. I wanted to manage this stage of my life naturally as opposed to taking medication. Reading more books and studies on natural remedies my curiosity about the journey of food throughout the ages, dietary changes and the many factors that influence how we eat grew. I soon realised that this was the option for me. The fascinating information I came across became the making of this book. I want to share this information with other men and women because, through research and conversations with my peers, what I discovered was that people were either oblivious to, or overwhelmed by, the volume of readily available information out there. This is one of the main reasons why I chose to write this book and embarked on studies in nutrition and personal development. Too much information can be confusing, and many of us are put off by this, especially when all we want to know are the facts and how we can improve our wellbeing.

Another issue that jumped out at me during my research was that men go through andropause, a transition similar to menopause, as they age. This made me sit up and take notice, as none of my male colleagues had ever mentioned it. Most of you have no doubt heard jokes of men reaching midlife and 'acting out', but nowhere had I read that men also go through The Change and, if left unchecked, it can lead to a host of health problems. Given this general lack of knowledge, I decided that it would be beneficial to include a chapter on this subject so that we could also improve the lives of our male counterparts. More information is emerging and I encourage men to take advantage of it and arm themselves with knowledge to improve their wellbeing.

Having concluded that we can make this transition less horrendous by changing our diet. I have put together information on supplements, herbs and vibrational foods, a menu plan and recipes to help balance your hormones to make this transition a smoother, less stressful experience.

CHAPTER 1

CHANGES BEFORE 'THE CHANGE'

So, you have reached the pinnacle of your career, more or less. Check. Your children are probably nearing the end of secondary school, at college or pretty much getting on with their lives. Check. You are in an established relationship, starting out in a new one or happily single. Check. You breathe a sigh of relief as you re-assess your life and tick off the boxes of your achievements. After all, you are in your late thirties or forties, and your life is how you planned it to be, or very nearly so. If it's not, you are probably thinking about what measures you can take to make life the way you want it. Now, you can focus on yourself as you relax in the knowledge that you have done as much as you can to set yourself up for your middle to senior years.

Hopefully, you are in good health or managing any ailments you might have. You would then be forgiven for missing the signs that The Change is upon you. The odd hot flash or two, the missed cycle, the irritability, the feelings of lethargy and low libido could be put down to feeling under the weather or the pressures of modern life, but what if they aren't? After all, most people tend to talk about the menopause happening to older people. Older peers or family members might have shared a horror story or two or maybe not. You may have even given it a fleeting thought but pushed it out of your head, thinking it was years away for you. Why think about it now? You probably believe menopause is for women in their later years, not you. You're not that old. You still have time.

Some of you may be experiencing symptoms right now, and the niggling doubts at the back of your mind might surface more often than you'd like to admit. But if you're like most people, you're in denial. You might have even wondered if you were going through the menopause, but let's back up just a little bit as there is one more change before The Change.

Drum roll, please…

Perimenopause.

Your body begins to prepare as early as 10 to 15 years before the onset of the menopause. Don't be caught off guard as I was. I pretty much ignored every symptom. Had I paid attention, I would have been more prepared for this phase of my life. Let's look at what our bodies go through during perimenopause.

The symptoms you might experience are similar to menopause, and that's where the confusion might lie for some of you. The first change is usually to your menstrual cycle: it may become irregular, have either a shorter or longer duration, be closer together, or be heavier or lighter. It may be spotty, or you might miss a period. If you are not pregnant, then it is likely that you are entering perimenopause. Palpitations are another symptom you might experience at this stage, and that can be quite frightening, to say the least. A racing heartbeat and fluttering sensations can leave you wondering if you are about to have a heart attack. This is caused by fluctuating hormone levels, particularly estrogen, which affects the mechanisms of the cardiovascular system. If you are concerned about your heart health, have a chat with your doctor or health practitioner, as this will enable you to rule out anything serious and put your mind at ease. I recall having bouts of palpitations when I went through this stage and having this symptom checked out at the hospital to find that nothing untoward was occurring with my heart, was much to my relief.

As estrogen levels decline, fluctuating hormones can not only affect other systems in the body, but they can also affect your oral health. Reports of periodontal disease and gingivitis are not uncommon in women as they enter perimenopause, as well as teeth discolouration and tooth loss. Being mindful about what you eat and speaking to your dentist about ways to manage your oral health during The Change is advisable to prevent tooth loss. We have enough to contend with as we go through this transition without having to worry about losing our pretty smiles. Being toothless can zap your confidence and body image.

Another symptom that can really knock your confidence is a loss of breast tissue caused by low progesterone levels. Your once perky breasts may now feel like empty sacs, or they will start to sag. Many women start to feel unattractive and unsexy, particularly in Western society, where voluptuous breasts are viewed as a symbol of sexiness. The rise in breast implants in midlife women shows the pressures that women are under to conform to this 'standard' of sexiness.

Other symptoms you may experience at this time include disruptive sleep patterns, fatigue, urine leakage when coughing or sneezing, the urgent need to urinate more frequently, discomfort during sex, a low libido and feelings of sadness or anger. These symptoms are caused by the effects of estrogen being out of balance, which affects the production of other hormones, such as serotonin.

Serotonin is a mood regulator. It declines simultaneously with the reduction in estrogen levels, causing symptoms of depression, anxiety and mood swings in the perimenopausal years. The term 'perimenopausal rage' is typical, and it plays out as feeling as cool as a cucumber one minute and then heightened anger or emotional outbursts the next. Your emotions will tend to swing as if on a pendulum as your hormones become more imbalanced. However, perimenopause and menopause are not a transition to fear as you enter mid-life. You can take back control of your body with a few measures to balance your hormones, so don't be disheartened. I will talk about this in detail, as well as other things you can do later on in this book, but first, let's look at the role of hormones.

CHAPTER 2

The Role of Hormones

The menopause presents women with many changes to their bodies as their sex hormones start powering down. Although you don't need to have a degree in hormone studies, having a basic understanding of their functions will help you make sense of symptoms you experience when perimenopause and menopause knock at your door. In this chapter, I dive into hormones to give you a snapshot of what's happening internally. From birth to pretty much into your 40s, your sex hormones generally work in harmony, running like a well-oiled machine unless you have a health condition that affects them. Your monthly cycle is regular like clockwork as long as your sex hormones work in synchronicity. If you struggle with your weight, changing your diet will generally help you achieve your desired weight goal. Your body is able to adjust to temperatures, burn calories efficiently, and, for the most part, you are able to deal with life challenges without getting too stressed unless there are areas in your life that create excess stress in the long term. It's not until your ovaries have reached the point of retirement that they become less responsive to controlling hormones released by the pituitary gland in the brain, and you start to notice subtle changes in your body and mood that generally increase over time. The most common change women notice is their mood and how they respond to everyday challenges. Situations they once found easy to manage or overlooked might become overwhelming. Moodiness and anxiety swiftly follow, and some women find it difficult to switch off, relax or get a good night's sleep. This usually happens when they experience a drop in progesterone. You may notice that you are easily irritated, snappy or zone out often. You may also experience poor quality sleep, wake up during the night and not be able to get back to sleep. I had many of these nights in perimenopause. Not having a good night's sleep affects other hormones like cortisol, which puts your body in a state of stress. Cortisol is your survival hormone. It prepares you for fight or flight, keeping you on the edge when it thinks you are under attack. Being in a state of perpetual readiness increases irritability, making it difficult for you to relax. When you can't unwind, you struggle to sleep, which has an impact on your energy levels, mood and concentration throughout the day. Being in constant survival mode can also cause hypertension. Needless to say, it's a vicious cycle, causing further frustration and anxiety. Many women in this state of despair consequently do not feel like themselves. I talk about how women feel about The Change and this new reality in later chapters.

Around this time, many women notice changes to their monthly cycle. Your cycle may become longer one month and shorter the next, heavier or lighter, as your estrogen levels fluctuate. Many women report having their first hot flashes, quickly followed by the onset of night sweats, which can cause embarrassing odour. I experienced night sweats for months that would disappear and return years later. I found that wearing layers often helped when I needed to cool down, and sleeping with the window ajar kept my bedroom cooler. Having good sleep hygiene is so important as symptoms can get really uncomfortable. Brain fog tends to go hand-in-hand with hot flashes, as does a lowered libido, as testosterone also dips in perimenopause. You may find that you lose your drive or spark and lack motivation. Procrastination is another symptom women complain about during this time. I spent a lot of money on products trying to get my drive back, not realising that the dip in hormones was the root cause. Hormone fluctuation can leave you feeling stressed and even fatigued, so don't be hard on yourself. Your mind and body need to adjust to this transition, so be gentle and show yourself compassion.

I won't repeat the laundry list of symptoms mentioned in Chapter 1; however, it would be remiss of me if I didn't mention the impact of menopause on a woman's looks. This symptom really deserves a separate chapter by itself, to be honest. Given that the beauty industry rakes in billions of pounds, I think it's important to have some understanding of how menopause can impact your looks and a few steps you can take now to minimise this impact. In my study of the menopause and its many impacts on the lives of women, I came across an article that referenced the *American Journal of Biological Anthropology* study on the ageing of male and female faces after andropause and menopause, respectively. The findings of this study noted that around the age of 50, the change or ageing rate of the face was more pronounced in women than in men. The journal also stated that aging was generally associated with a flatter face, sagged soft tissue, deeper creases in the skin extending from both sides of your nose to the corners of your mouth, thinner lips and longer nose and ears (Windhager et al., 2019). These changes were brought on by the decline in collagen levels, particularly in the skin and bone of the face. Also, subcutaneous fat, which is the fat just below your skin, plays a pivotal role in shaping facial contour, with women experiencing unevenly distributed subcutaneous fat around the cheek area and muscle loss in the face

Changes in facial appearance occurring with the menopause can be distressing and severely affect one's self-confidence and quality of life. Needless to say, internally, there is a lot happening as you navigate the menopause. If you want to slow down this process, I suggest finding ways to help your body produce more collagen. There are simple things you can do, such as taking a collagen supplements or consume bone broth regularly. Collagen supplements may help with elasticity in your skin and give your skin a glow. Do some research into different ones before buying, as not all do as they say on the label. If you don't want to consume animal products, increase your intake of plant-based foods rich in vitamin C, zinc and copper to help your body boost collagen production. Copper is a mineral that slows down the ageing process and helps with bone density and holding connective tissue together. Copper is also beneficial for thyroid health. Foods rich in copper are liver, kidney, shellfish, sesame seeds and shitake mushrooms (West, 2023). Some professionals tout the benefits of using copper utensils (Patil, 2022). I recently purchased a copper water bottle, so I'm keeping a watchful eye on my appearance for evidence of its effectiveness. Needless to say, there is a lot happening inside your body; if you experience this transition with minimal symptoms, you are very fortunate.

By now, you will have gathered that hormones are quintessential to the health and function of our bodies in a variety of ways. Made up of amines, peptides and proteins, the majority of these chemical messengers are housed in the endocrine system and are released through major glands: pituitary, pineal, thymus, thyroid, adrenal, pancreas, testes and ovaries. Blood carries these hormones to organs and tissues to exert functions such as development and growth, metabolism of food, sexual function, reproductive growth and health, cognitive function, maintenance of body temperature, thirst, sleep, digestion and much more. On a psychological level, hormones have an impact on our cognitive function, mood, behaviour and even attraction. Yes, even attraction. Apparently, hormones are responsible for the chemistry of love that helps you form and maintain romantic connections, which are deepened by oxytocin. Estrogen and testosterone also play a role in the chemistry of love. Estrgoen, directly affects oxytocin levels and helps with regulating arousal, and testosterone plays a role in boosting libido. Can you now see why a woman's sex drive might nose-dive in menopause? According to research carried out by *AARP*, men blame lack of sex as the leading reason for divorce in midlife (Montenegro, 2004, p. 204). Evidently, a lack of intimacy can be linked to your hormones. Medication can also have an impact on intimacy, such as the ones you take for allergies and hypertension. It is worth noting here that if you are genuinely happy in singledom, then this area of your life will not be an issue; however, if you are concerned about intimacy, speak to your doctor or health coach. Don't suffer in silence. There could be herbs, supplements or medication that can help get your mojo back.

When looking at the menopause, most of the focus has been on estrogen, progesterone and testosterone, as these are the main hormones that work in concert to develop sex characteristics and reproductive cycles. However, they do exert influence on other hormones, causing a range of emotional and physical shifts when levels dip, as you have just read about when it comes to romantic connections. Many women say they just don't feel like themselves anymore and experience bouts of feeling overwhelmed, poor concentration or sadness that start creeping in around the time of The Change. Some women disclose that they lack an interest in activities they once found rewarding or they find life lacklustre. You might be surprised to learn that estrogen has a direct impact on dopamine and serotonin levels, which are reward neurotransmitters, your feel-good hormones, responsible for emotional and motivational behaviours such as pleasure, motivation, learning and decision-making. (Cleveland Clinic, 2023). Consequently, a dip in estrogen can lead to dopamine and serotonin deficiency. If you find that you lack motivation, have lost your spark/mojo, become forgetful, feel hopeless or have restless nights, it's quite possible that your dopamine level is low. It is then not surprising to learn that women going through menopause are at an increased risk of anxiety and depression, given the role of estrogen on dopamine in maintaining its activity. In fact, some experts believe that changes in dopamine activity might contribute to certain schizophrenic symptoms. Antipsychotic medicine for this type of mental illness is a dopamine-serotonin stabiliser, demonstrating the vital role these hormones play in your overall emotional well-being and mental health.

So, what is the link between menopause and mental illness?

When looking through records in doctors' offices and hospitals, a London scientist noticed that a lot of women were being diagnosed with schizophrenia after the age of 45. Historically, this diagnosis had not been given to women over the age of 40. Consequently, some women experiencing mental illness during menopause might actually be misdiagnosed. There are limited studies on this, according to the article I read on the Healthy Women website (Kraft, 2019). It noted that a deficiency in dopamine can be a catalyst in women with an underlying risk for schizophrenia or other mental illnesses.

There's so much to consider when going through the menopause. The loss of our precious sex hormones can have an impact on us in so many ways. However, it must be noted that although our ovaries produce most of these hormones, our adrenals and fat tissue also produce the hormone pregnenolone, a precursor for cortisol, estrogen, testosterone and progesterone. The primary role of our adrenal glands is to help us manage daily stress through the production of adrenaline, our fight or flight reaction to threats, and cortisol, our body's main stress hormone. It's really imperative that you manage your stress load, as cumulative stress and anxiety can deplete your adrenals. This occurs when your adrenals increase cortisol production to help your body cope with the extra demand as it believes your body is under threat. This takes away from the production of pregnenolone that would normally go into making sex hormones, primarily progesterone, boosting cortisol instead. Sleepless nights, palpitations, urinary incontinence, low libido, stiff and/or painful joints and weight gain, particularly in the midriff, are signs that your adrenals are struggling. High-stress levels may also cause estrogen dominance, which not only has a knock-on effect on your adrenals but also on your thyroid and norepinephrine, a hormone and neurotransmitter produced by the brain and adrenals in periods of stress or excitement. Just to note, a serotonin deficiency can also increase norepinephrine levels, which has a knock-on effect on the hypothalamic thermostat, which can trigger hot flashes and night sweats. We don't hear much about norepinephrine, but it shows up a lot on the bioresonance scans I carry out as a part of the Body MOT in my mobile health practice. In it, you can see the effect of one hormone upon others. Given the functions of the adrenals, looking after them during menopause should be your priority for your overall health and well-being. Herbs such as ashwagandha and holy basil support adrenal health, lower cortisol and support the healthy functions of norepinephrine. You can find more herbs to help you manage menopause symptoms as you read through this book.

Hormones are super-powerful and have complex interrelationships. A deficiency in one hormone can have an impact on another, and too much or too little of a particular hormone can have very serious health consequences. There is a hormone that produces symptoms mimicking menopausal symptoms if you have too much or too little. Let's look at the thyroid, a small, butterfly-shaped gland in your neck that plays an important role in regulating your body's metabolism.

Excessive estrogen can cause an enlarged thyroid or underactive thyroid function. If your thyroid is underactive, you may experience symptoms similar to menopause, such as hot flashes, insomnia, palpitations, dry skin, weight gain, fatigue, poor concentration and brain fog. Apparently, up to 20% of women have underactive thyroid function (Miller & Seegert, 2025. An overactive thyroid, known as hyperthyroidism, can include symptoms such as weight loss, irritability and tiredness. This is because estrogen and thyroid hormones play a pivotal role in bone structure, body thermostat regulation, mood, metabolism and the rate at which your body converts food to energy. If you experience any of these symptoms, you might want to have your thyroid and iodine levels checked. Iodine is an important mineral for thyroid function, particularly for your metabolic rate, and this is super important in menopause, given the impact of estrogen on thyroid function and the impact it can have on your weight, skin, hair, health and emotions. You can generally help your thyroid by including iodine-rich foods like sea moss, kelp, oysters, eggs, sardines and foods rich in selenium, such as Brazil nuts, in your diet (Zhou et al., 2016) and reducing processed and refined foods.

Weight gain is a topic that often comes up in conversation in my friendship circle, as some of us have gone up a dress size or more since starting menopause. We share our struggles about trying to lose belly fat and the many diets and other things we have tried to get back to our pre-menopausal weight. A few had other health problems, which, upon further investigation, found were markers of metabolic syndrome.

Metabolic syndrome consists of a cluster of risk factors that increase the risk of type 2 diabetes and cardiovascular disease. This cluster includes dysglycemia, increased blood pressure, lipid abnormalities as defined by hypertriglyceridemia and low high-density lipoprotein cholesterol, and central obesity, known as visceral fat (Meyer et al. 2011). This type of fat is stored around the midsection of your body behind the abdominal muscles. This happens during menopause due to hormone imbalances when body fat tends to shift to the abdomen. A small amount is fine as it protects the organs; however, having more visceral fat is linked to higher risk of chronic diseases.

Given that I was at risk for this syndrome, I had to have a plan of action to improve my health. The signs were there, and I had to act fast, given that I had visceral fat and my blood pressure was just above the range of average. Armed with the findings of my health audit and the knowledge from the chef's course I was studying, I started to make small changes, such as swapping out croissants and tea for fruit salad and yoghurt for breakfast and increasing my protein intake. Not being one for the gym, daily walks became my routine to lose some of the extra pounds I had gained in recent years as I was not as active as I used to be, and my hormones were fluctuating. The pounds are now dropping off, which is a confidence boost.

Changing my diet wasn't as hard as I thought it would be. I hit a few blocks at the start as I was an emotional eater, and I had formed some unhealthy eating habits, primarily snacking when bored or stressed, so I had to work on my relationship with food. Studying as a natural chef, a course that focused on the energetics of foods and herbs, helped me deal with my food challenges as well as stabilise my hormones. I cover diet and nutrition for hormone health in later chapters, which will help you make more positive food choices to manage menopausal symptoms.

It is no secret that we have become a nation of couch potatoes. You only have to turn on the news or read health publications to know that obesity is on the increase in middle-aged men and women. We are not as active as we were in our younger years, and a lot more of us have been working from home since the pandemic, which makes for a more sedentary lifestyle. Couple this with a diet of high fat and sugar intake, and we end up on a trajectory to type 2 diabetes, which is a marker of metabolic syndrome. According to a study carried out by the University of Glasgow, people of Asian, Black African and Caribbean ethnicities have been found to be two to four times more likely to have diabetes than white populations (Ntuk et al., 2013). I am not surprised by their findings, as Caribbean and Asian diets consist largely of proteins and white rice. White rice is a starch with a high glycaemic load, which can spike your blood sugar levels. You might be surprised to learn that a diet of refined foods can spike blood sugar levels as well as trigger the menopause one-and-a-half years earlier than average, (Cade et al, 2018).

If you are concerned about diabetes, start keeping a food diary to get a snapshot of your diet. It's so easy in today's fast-paced society to get breakfast on the go if you're not working from home. Grabbing a coffee and toast, a croissant or a muffin for breakfast can often put stress on your pancreas's ability to produce insulin, and convert glucose into energy. If you notice that your diet primarily consists of processed and refined foods, consider cutting back. Consume more low glycaemic foods to help blood glucose levels, like oatmeal. Adding selenium-rich foods to your diet, like Brazil nuts and yams, is also a great way to help with insulin sensitivity.

There are so many things that can have an impact on our hormones as we go through the menopause, and it is easy to miss the root cause of some of the symptoms, particularly weight gain. It wasn't until I purchased the bioresonance scan for my practice that I became aware of the roles of leptin and ghrelin. These hormones are responsible for your appetite, and an imbalance can cause you to overeat. Leptin signals to your body that you are full, so you don't overeat, and ghrelin signals to your body that you are hungry. If your leptin is dysregulated, your brain will not receive the signal that you have just eaten; therefore, you might find that you are often hungry throughout the day, which can result in you gaining excessive weight as you eat more to subdue hunger pangs. The primary factors disrupting ghrelin are stress, not getting enough sleep and blood sugar levels, as ghrelin is regulated by the body's circadian rhythm or biological clock. Getting a good night's sleep helps regulate the production of these two hormones. This made sense to me as, during the time of my weight gain, I did not prioritise sleep, and I was often in stress mode due to a lot of demands on my time. To say that I needed a life overhaul when I was transitioning into the menopause would be an understatement.

Paying particular attention to factors that can affect the function of hormones is important as our bodies go through perimenopause and menopause, and there are many factors that influence it. Simple tasks we do on a daily basis can throw our hormones into disarray. For example, many cleaning products contain chemicals that are endocrine disruptors. Glycol ethers are chemicals present in some household products, like paints and cleaning products, that disrupt your hormones. Chemical compounds used to make plastics flexible and lubricants in personal care products like phthalates are often referred to as endocrine disruptors. We drink out of plastic bottles that contain BPA, a known carcinogen that sucks away testosterone and can cause infertility. It's great to see that some manufacturers are being responsible and producing BPA-free plastic bottles. You may also be surprised to learn that some cosmetic products are made with ingredients that can have an impact on your hormones, like formaldehyde, lead, oxybenzone, and more. Even chemicals we put on our hair can affect our hormones. The rise in non-chemically produced makeup and beauty products is the beauty industry's response to these growing health concerns. Beauty is becoming a costly business, not just financially, but to our health as well.

It's not only what we put on our skin that affects our hormones, but what we eat.

Certain foods can interfere with our hormones. Let's look at chicken, for example. Chicken is the preferred protein option over red meat because of the public's awareness of the amount of saturated fat in red meat. However, like livestock, non-organic chickens are given antibiotics and synthetic hormones regularly to ensure rapid development, increased muscle mass and to keep them as healthy as possible given their cramped living conditions in concentrated animal feed operations

(CAFOs). However, the excessive hormones and antibiotics in meat can disrupt our hormone levels, particularly estrogen, the hormone promoting and maintaining female characteristics in the body, like the menstrual cycle, sexual development, pregnancy, childbirth and the onset of menopause.

The rise in pescatarians is likely a consequence of the concerns around meat production and the care of animals. However, consuming more fish, which is seen as a healthier option over meat may not be as healthy as you assumed as it depends on where fish is sourced. Fish are particularly loaded with PCBs and mercury, two very powerful hormone disruptors, and the larger the fish, the more of these chemicals they contain. Other foods that can contribute to hormone disruption are processed high-fat, high-carbohydrate foods like pastries, chips, fried foods, white rice and bread, according to Dr. Christiane Northrup, a physician and author of *The Wisdom of Menopause* (2012). Most bread products contain added gluten in addition to the naturally occurring gluten in wheat. Gluten and sugar increase inflammation production in the body which, in turn, places stress on the adrenal glands, affecting the thyroid, gonads and autoimmunity, consequently reducing their ability to produce hormones. Furthermore, consuming too much sugar can cause an imbalance in sex hormones, estrogen, progesterone and testosterone, because your body prioritises balancing insulin levels over producing these hormones.

When we think about the many ways in which we can disrupt our hormones, we would be forgiven for feeling overwhelmed. Many of the products we use are regulated; however, some of the chemicals may not appear on the packaging, so it's difficult to know what's contained in the product. In addition, regulators do not take into consideration the cumulative effect of using several products daily or eating the same nutrient-poor products consistently. Educating yourself on your diet as you transition into perimenopause is super important.

So, what can you do to help your hormones, given the quintessential roles they play?

- Consume organic foods and pasture-raised animal products. Organic food has more of the nutrients the body needs than non-organic food because the soil it is grown in has not been depleted by over-farming and harmful agricultural practices.

- Start using natural products on your skin as these are mainly free from harmful chemicals, irritants and preservatives.

- Reduce your exposure to BPA, a known carcinogen, by drinking out of glass bottles instead of plastic bottles and storing food in glass containers.

- Avoid warming food in plastic containers in the microwave. Instead, microwave food in glass or ceramic containers.

- Replace plastic housewares labelled 'microwave-safe' if they have been scratched or if the colour has changed, as chemicals can potentially leach into your food.

As you read on, you will learn about ways to manage your hormones as you go through perimenopause and menopause and other ways of improving emotional and physiological health and well-being. Managing hormones should not be limited to people of a certain age. It's never too early to start making lifestyle changes.

CHAPTER 3

The Seasoned Woman

reached that stage in my life with very little knowledge of The Change, and I was none the wiser after speaking to women who seemed to have survived menopause unscathed or had blotted the experience from their minds. The few women prepared to discuss their transition to menopause filled my mind with horror stories of ravaging symptoms that plagued them for months, even years: hair loss, burning hands and feet, dry, itchy eyes and sweaty scalp. Needless to say, fear engulfed my mind. I spent countless hours looking into the menopause and what it meant for women, and I decided to share what I learnt with you so you won't feel as confused as I did.

So, here goes...

Menopause is a natural transition that every woman experiences. The symptoms vary, and every woman's experience is different to some degree. It has been described as puberty in reverse due to the decline in sexual reproduction and the changes it brings to your body, similar to how puberty brought changes many years ago. Your ovaries are going into retirement, producing fewer hormones, and you are more reliant on the adrenals to take over estrogen production; granted, it won't be to the same extent as your ovaries. Consequently, you will be left with less estrogen and likely many symptoms. If you have not read the previous chapter on hormones, read it before continuing with this chapter, as having an awareness of hormonal changes will help you understand what could be happening to your body.

The age of onset for menopause is typically around 51. This is when estrogen levels start to decline shortly after a dip in progesterone, which triggers perimenopause. However, it must be noted that treatment for certain conditions or illnesses, such as cancer or a full hysterectomy, can throw you into menopause much earlier. This is known as surgical or induced menopause. Your doctor may encourage you to take hormone replacement therapy (HRT) and testosterone medication until you reach the average age that menopause occurs, to help with cognitive function and reduce the risk of osteoporosis and cardiovascular disease. In 2025, an estimated 1.1 billion women worldwide are in menopause (Astellas, 2024). That's a large section of the population going through this transition at the same time.

So, what can you expect?

There are three hormonal stages women experience throughout their lives: premenopause, perimenopause and menopause. In short, the premenopausal phase is the child bearing stage, when periods are regular and sometimes accompanied by cramps, anxiety, mood swings, irritability and nausea. Most women transition from this stage to perimenopause in their 40s. The primary indicator of entering this second phase is often irregular periods and severe mood swings. Once a woman has reached the menopause, she will have regular occurrences of symptoms associated with perimenopause with only one difference: No periods for 12 months. The intensity of symptoms will reduce within the first few years when symptoms begin to reduce as the body stabilises. However, the risk of coronary heart disease, osteoporosis and endometrial cancer increases due to producing less of those precious sex hormones. As women live longer, the average woman can spend over one-third of her life — that's an awful lot of time functioning on a reduction of these special hormones. I recall conversations with my friends about our exasperation and frustration with night sweats and hot flashes, duvet on, duvet off, on and off for hours during the night. Window open, window closed. My partner at the time thought I was losing the plot. He was much younger and did not understand anything about the change of life women go through other than that it was experienced by old people. What a cheek!

It was the middle of winter when I had my first hot flash. I was at my desk and felt a sudden surge of heat rush through my body. I thought someone had ramped up the heat after all the complaints about how cold the office had been all week. Sweat trickled down my back, and I loosened the top buttons on my blouse, removed my jacket, grabbed a report off my desk and began to fan myself, ignoring the odd looks from my colleagues. I thought I was coming down with a virus, maybe the flu, but within minutes, it had gone. I felt the chill of the office and quickly put my jacket back on. The hot flash was soon forgotten as I became absorbed in my work. It was months later before I had another hot flash, the frequency of which only increased over the subsequent weeks. Feeling like an overheated radiator during the day soon transitioned into a nighttime occurrence. Night sweats, is characterised by sudden, intense heat, perspiration, heart palpitations, nausea, headaches, flushing, chills and interrupted sleep. This happens due to the drop in estrogen, which fools your body into thinking you are overheating. If you've had them before, you will know how uncomfortable hot flashes and night sweats can be. It feels as though you are sitting in front of a blazing fireplace dressed in woollens, gloves and a hat and someone has blasted the heater to 90 degrees. It makes you want to jump out of your skin. The sudden heat or redness often starts in the face, neck or chest and spreads, making you sweat. An increased heart rate and palpitations are commonly associated with hot flashes. Waking up with the bedclothes drenched in sweat is uncomfortable and exasperating because you can't go back to sleep in a wet bed, and changing sheets at 3 a.m is no fun. Up to 80% of midlife women experience hot flashes at some point in this transition (Gallicchio et al., 2015). Hot flashes are most frequent and intense during the first two years of the menopause when estrogen levels drop below a certain point.

Another source of frustration for women going through the menopause is the change in skin texture. Gone is the soft, plump, smooth skin and in its place is decreased skin thickness and elasticity, dryness, depigmentation and the loss of collagen as estrogen levels reduce. Your youthful face may now be lax and lined with crow's feet around the eyes and deep line around the corner of your mouth or eyes. I talk about facial changes in Chapter 2. If you missed it, go back and have a read as I share some really good tips to slow down the ageing of your skin. The products used prior to the menopause often fail to support the skin. I dread to think how much money I spent trying to find suitable skincare products allegedly designed for ageing and menopausal skin. My skin is very sensitive and easily irritated; I now use grapeseed oil and castor oils as they suit my skin better, and I have managed to create a blend that's perfect for me. You might find that you have to shop around (I did), but it's worth it to get skincare products that work best for you. Calling this *The Change* is apt as we may morph into people we hardly recognise. Weight gain, hair loss or excessive hair growth on the face, the loss of libido, and not feeling attractive or overlooked are some reasons women give for letting themselves go or contemplating cosmetic surgery. Given the symptoms I listed above, you would be hard-pressed to view menopause as a positive transition. What's even more frustrating is that many doctors and gynaecologists are not trained in menopausal care and, therefore, offer very little in the way of support to women who might approach them for help. This is one of the primary reasons why I wrote this book. I hope you feel more empowered as you read on.

Are there some benefits to the menopause?

In some instances, menopause is welcomed. I had fibroids that caused painful menstruation and heavy bleeding, which I later found out from a naturopathic therapist, were caused by estrogen-dominance triggered by my diet. The cessation of my monthly cycle was a relief. Those damn fibroids had caused me nothing but problems because the bulky growths pressed on my bladder, and I was forever running to the loo. I was frustrated, to say the least. Bloating, irritability, being highly sensitive, and the chocolate cravings and brain fog I experienced on the days leading up to my period definitely will not be missed. I love chocolate, menses or not, but I really don't miss having to wear a tampon or a sanitary towel. What an inconvenience. I also don't miss the many embarrassing accidents I had when I leaked on to my clothes. For me, the menopause is freedom from all that. I have become more balanced and finally have the time to focus on myself. Doing inner work and re-examining my roles has given me a new lease on life. And there is no more risk of getting pregnant or being concerned about birth control. I have developed a whole new level of confidence as I re-awaken passions that have lain dormant whilst raising my family. More about that later.

Menopause often triggers major changes in the brain through neural plasticity, a kind of rewiring that can also lead to deep spiritual shifts. Hailed as the ending by many in Western society, the menopause is actually viewed as a new beginning in some cultures. Granted, the menopause can be an ordeal and a downright terrible experience, and I am not playing down the symptoms. Your body has changed and does not function the way it used to. You can almost feel like your body has been taken over by an outside entity. Many women are unprepared for the physical and psychological changes that come with perimenopause and menopause at a time when women are likely to be facing additional challenges. Some of these challenges can relate to finances and the anxiety of not having enough for retirement. According to a study by Investec Wealth & Retirement (U.K.), a part of the Rathbones Group, approximately 56% of women are concerned that they are not financially prepared for retirement. The group advises women to speak to a financial advisor about options (Brately, 2024). Caring for ageing parents can also present many challenges, particularly if you are still in full-time employment, live far away from your parents or have additional commitments. The pressure of juggling many hats at this time or role overload, as it is often termed, has seen many women buckle under the strain of the demand. Becoming an empty-nester is another huge adjustment and shock to many women who find that they now have many hours to fill as they are no longer caring for their children. This may sound like a dream to most of us, but to some, it can actually feel like a nightmare. Some women talk about the void that comes with being an empty nester and the wave of sadness and anxiety they experience as they grieve the loss of how things used to be and have to adjust to a new reality, which is often lonely. I felt alone for many years after my children left home. Although I saw them often, it was difficult for me to adjust to not being needed as much. I did, however, adjust after a while, and I now enjoy a new level of freedom. I now embrace being an empty nester and exploring new opportunities. It is a great time to take a life inventory/audit to assess and do an overhaul or reboot, in a sort of decluttering or shedding of things, even if it is with people who no longer add value to your life. If you are a Bible reader, you have likely come across this scripture in Ecclesiastes 3 verse 6 that encourages us to declutter. It states that there is 'a time to keep, and a time to cast away.' If something or someone no longer serves you, why hang on to it or them? I often repeated the words 'less is more' sometimes daily when I was overwhelmed and needed not only to clear my mind, but also my home. I now embrace a more minimalist lifestyle. According to Maria (2019), founder of the organisation Dare to Declutter, the act of decluttering is a therapeutic journey, helping you let go of the past, make room for the present, and embrace a more mindful future. Decluttering can also be a way to clear the way for a new YOU!

The menopause can be a time of rebirth in which you give birth to the real you. I see it as a time for you to live up to your true potential. Spiritually, it is a time of exciting change and new beginnings, a time to heal old wounds caused by losses you might have carried for far too long. It is a time for soul care. The energy you once dedicated to others is now yours to use on you. As a woman's estrogen level reduces, she can become more self-absorbed or self-full. Embracing the opportunity to really listen to their bodies, noticing the subtle and not so subtle changes, gives women the chance to go within and become more aware of their bodies and their needs. Spiritually, it is a time to focus on self-fulfilment. Unfortunately, this experience can be undermined by the negative view of menopause in Western society that women buy into, whereby ageing and menopause are not viewed as positive. On a deeper level, denying the healing of old wounds, which is often expressed as stagnation and limitation, results in unfulfilled dreams and passions. In our youth-idolising culture, the menopause is often seen as an ending. Women are often mocked by their female co-workers or friends when they experience hot flashes, memory loss, brain fog, verbal slips or other obvious cognitive effects brought about by perimenopause and menopause. It disturbs me that women can treat their peers in this way, even more so, as these symptoms can contribute to the reasons why many women give up their jobs because they simply cannot manage in the workplace anymore. Up to one-third of women struggle at work due to menopause, according to studies (D'Angelo, 2022). It is promising that employers across the country are developing menopause policies to support women, given that lost productivity as a result of the menopause costs U.K. companies billions of pounds each year. Having a workplace policy is a positive step in the right direction to support women in midlife who make up a large section of the workforce.

Menopause is a new landscape for women in this century as we are living longer and, therefore, spending more years in menopause than women a century ago. The natural lifespan for women back then was 57 years old (central statistical release 2020), which meant that they did not spend too much time in menopause. Given that menopause has been shrouded in secrecy for so long, I dread to imagine what women went through even a decade ago when menopause was still taboo. Conversations about menopause are much needed today, as there is still so much to learn about this transition.

In other parts of the world, women are honoured at this time of life. Mayan women look forward to this transition and view it as a time of newfound freedom and status. They are often held in high regard in their communities as spiritual leaders or wise women (Tait, 2022). Asian women are also valued as wise women in their communities. In Japan, the word for menopause is *konenki*, which means renewal and regeneration (Women's Health Network, 2013). This is such a positive outlook. I, too, view menopause as a renewal, a second spring, a time to redefine yourself or have a rebirth, as it can open so many doors if you shift your mindset to one that is positive and embracing. Some studies reveal that a positive attitude can reduce the severity of some menopause symptoms (Bień, 2024). Why not make a list of all the positives now that you are in menopause? The cessation of monthly periods is at the top of my list. Prioritising me is a close second.

I am often encouraged when I meet women in midlife who 'keep it together', refusing to let misconceptions like women in midlife are unhappy, uninteresting and unsexy hold them back and are taking charge of their lives instead, creating new and exciting experiences. If nothing else, this should give you the inspiration to embrace the transition and see it as a new and exhilarating chapter in your life. We have powerful women like Kathie Lee Gifford (who is a well-known actress and producer) and Naomi Campbell (an iconic supermodel who still walks runways in her 50s) who are likely to be perimenopausal or in menopause. There are also many women running major companies across the globe, like Raksha Shah, who started her nutrition business at 65. In fact, there are many midlife founders starting new careers who are likely in the throes of menopause, who don't allow this transition to hinder their careers. Going back to early recorded history, there are amazing accounts of women in the Bible who were considered wise and instrumental. There was Deborah (who was a prophet and a judge) and Naomi (who nurtured and guided her daughter-in-law Ruth) who, when Ruth's husband died, which was likely when she was in midlife and possibly perimenopausal, went on to marry a wealthy prince. So, ladies, if you are still waiting for your prince, don't give up hope. He might be around the corner. The notion that menopausal women are redundant is outdated and challenged by these women and many more, and not a moment too soon, in my opinion.

You are a seasoned woman with various skills, experiences and knowledge which you can use to help others and younger women, too. Gone are the days of vulnerability and insecurity, you are blessed with a level of emotional stability accumulated after years of problem-solving and overcoming adversity and are unapologetically you. You can now embrace menopause and let it be the catalyst for a new beginning and increase your faith if you shift your mindset from one of lack to one of abundance. As you read on, you will discover how to adjust to your new identity as a woman in menopause, a period described by some as shifting sands. But first, let's look at our male counterparts and what they might experience during midlife.

CHAPTER 4

The Seasoned Man

Researching the andropause, the male equivalent to the menopause, was not as straightforward as I imagined, primarily due to the limited information available. This is in stark contrast to information available on the menopause, which is universal and well-characterised. In any event, it was a useful exercise as it demonstrated that society does not give this subject the attention it deserves, nor does it want to portray men as lacking in virility. I recently read an article in the local *Metro Newspaper* on my journey to work about the andropause, known as the forgotten epidemic. It was an interesting article, and the author effectively highlighted the fact most men who are experiencing this condition are suffering in silence due to a lack of knowledge about the andropause. This is quite alarming and concerning as, like women, men also experience changes to their bodies because of hormonal imbalances (Macrae, 2011). However, according to this article these symptoms were not being fully investigated. I am pleased that information about the andropause is now getting some press coverage and that men now have a term of reference for symptoms that might be afflicting them daily.

Researching the andropause was quite edifying. I was surprised to discover that, similar to their female counterparts, men also have hormonal cycles. 'A study of young men showed that the majority had a discernible cycle of testosterone with repeating rises and falls, but each man who did show a cycle had a cycle unique to himself' (Diamond, 2012). Men's hormone cycles fluctuate throughout the year. In studies conducted in the United States, France, and Australia, it was found that men secrete their highest levels of sex hormones in October and their lowest levels in April. There was a 16% increase in testosterone levels from April to October and a 22% decline from October to April. Interestingly, although Australia, for example, is in its springtime when France and the United States are in their autumn, men in all three parts of the world showed a similar pattern of peaks in October and valleys in April. (Diamond, 2012) According to Dr Diamond, a member of the International Scientific Board of the World Congress on Men's Health: When a man is asleep, his testosterone levels rise hour by hour until by the time he awakens, he is at his highest (morning erection). By the early and late morning, their levels typically level off and begin to decline. (2012)

So, what happens to men's hormones as they age?

Let us look more at the andropause. The name 'andropause' comes from the Greek *andro* (man) and *pauser* or *pausare* (to halt or cease) and was first coined in the 1940s. For centuries, it was dismissed by the medical community and often seen as an excuse for men to engage in uncharacteristic behaviours or 'behave badly', such as buying fast cars and motorbikes, spending copious amounts of time on computer games or chasing after young women. Consequently, to this day, a lot of men think that 'male menopause' is merely a myth. Andropause is a social taboo, and rather than discuss this issue openly, most men 'suck up and put up' by virtue of their masculinity, in contrast to their female counterparts. I broached this subject with a few of my male friends to gauge their knowledge on the andropause and was met with looks of shock and disdain. The idea of men going through The Change was unthinkable to them. Their response confirmed to me that more discussion needed to be had on this subject.

It is possible that men are typically disinclined to disclose any psychological or sexual failings and may not pay too much attention to physiological changes in their bodies as they grow older because of the pressure of modern society. This 'masculine gold standard' prizes power, control and invincibility. The truth, however, is that male menopause is real, and leaving it unchecked increases the risk of being stricken with certain cardiovascular, reproductive and other systemic diseases that typically come with age.

I was staggered to learn that the andropause affects one in five men over 50, that's approximately 2 million Brits alone, but only about 1% are ever diagnosed and treated (Morrison, 2024). Symptoms are not too dissimilar from those experienced by women going through menopause: joint pain, low libido, low mood, depression, poor concentration, irritability, weight gain, hot flashes, loss of muscle mass, fatigue and osteoporosis. Osteoporosis can shorten the spinal column (Mayo Clinic, 2022) (apparently, that's why their pants get too long). Additionally, they can experience erectile dysfunction, enlarged breasts, reduction in body and facial hair, and reduction in speed and duration (Mayo Clinic, 2022). Unlike women, symptoms in men are more gradual and can last longer. And just like menopause, andropause is caused by a hormonal imbalance or deficiency.

Healthy men can still be fertile well into their 80s and even later because the testes never totally run out of the substance they need to produce testosterone. Similar to the menopause in women, the andropause can be likened to reverse puberty. This transition can wreak havoc on men's social, interpersonal, psychological, sexual and spiritual wellbeing (Schwarz et al., 2011) as testosterone declines. This has an impact on energy levels, resulting in irritability, depression and lack of interest in sex. Your go-getter partner may become nonchalant, lacking drive and enthusiasm as their zest for life diminishes. Couples going through The Change at the same time are likely to find this period trying and testing to say the least. Addressing the root cause, which is a hormonal imbalance, becomes more of a necessity at this time to reduce the challenges these transitions presents to both of you.

It is crucial, then, that men are more informed about the changes going on inside their bodies as they age. They are encouraged to get their testosterone levels checked if they are concerned about symptoms associated with the andropause. A simple blood test will help diagnose this condition and is the first step to finding suitable treatment. Leaving it unchecked increases the risk that they will fall prey to cardiovascular, reproductive and other systemic diseases that usually come with age. Making healthy lifestyle choices, such as improving diet, can have a huge impact on relieving andropause symptoms. Regular exercise can also help in this regard, as it may improve testosterone levels, muscle mass concentration, mood and sleep.

Given that these changes can affect a man's emotional wellbeing and challenge to his sense of self, maybe, one day, the World Health Organization will have a designated day for the andropause as they do for the menopause. Until such time, men as well as women might want to consider how they are going to manage their respective transitions. Diet plays a major role in how we experience The Change. I explore the role of nutrition in more detail in subsequent chapters.

CHAPTER 5

The Black Woman's Experience

One thing for certain is that all women go through the menopause, and some of us find this transition much easier than others for various reasons. Having read thus far, you will hopefully be empowered to know there are simple steps you can start making to change your diet and lifestyle to have a better menopause experience. So, why are things generally different for Black women? To my knowledge, we all function the same unless I missed something significant in Biology class. Thankfully, that was not the case. I won't go into genetics here that's another book… maybe.

An article that I read about how Black women disproportionately experience menopause piqued my interest. It was written by Sheila Eldred (2023) and published in *Sahan Journal*. The article explored the impact of structural racism and other cultural and societal factors that contribute to Black women's experience of the menopause. After reading this article and coming across similar findings to what I now view as an understudied area of the menopause, I thought it of great importance to share this knowledge to raise awareness when it comes to Black women's experience. Please read this chapter with an open mind. Take each point as not being set in stone but as an opportunity to explore further, as we are still really learning about the menopause, given that it is not a topic that has been discussed openly until recently. To say that the possibility other groups might experience this transition differently was something I had limited knowledge of.

As a Wellness Practitioner, specialising in the menopause, I have advised Black women who reached out to me about uncomfortable symptoms from which they desperately wanted relief, like hot flashes, night sweats, palpitations, tinnitus and vertigo that were enough to disrupt their day at times. Some of these symptoms, as I recently found out, are experienced more intensely by Black women than other groups, according to research. One client I worked with was seriously considering leaving her job of 20 years because she felt unable to function at work due to frequent palpitations and vertigo. Thankfully, she has an understanding manager who allowed her to work from home most of the week. In fact, this new work from home culture has probably helped a lot of women going through menopause because it gives them more control over their environment. At home, you can adjust the temperature, open a window or wear what you want to stay cool during hot flashes, or you can lie down until the vertigo wears off. Being able to work from home occasionally when I was in the full throes of menopause was a godsend, so long may this arrangement continue, I say.

Back to the findings: The article references a study carried out by SWAN, an organisation that examines the physical, biological, psychological and social changes during this transitional period that has been studying racial disparities in menopause since the mid-90s, (Faubion et al., 2023). The study found that Black women tended to start menopause earlier than women from other groups and had more intense and frequent symptoms, such as hot flashes and night sweats. Furthermore, Black women endure these symptoms far longer than other groups. The study explained that cumulative stress was the primary reason for Black women's experience, caused by systemic racism. I was taken aback by this finding. I had to pause to reflect on what was new information to me. Not only does racism cause stress and anxiety, but it also has wider repercussions, namely a knock-on effect on your hormones. This appears to be largely overlooked in a lot of material about menopause, so I was keen to learn more about it.

Another study that shares similar findings is the American one by the Fawcett Society and Runnymede Trust, which looked into how women experienced racism (Gyimah et al., 2022). In their study, they discovered that 75% of Black women experienced racism at work. Although it is widely reported that women generally face a glass ceiling when applying for senior positions within the workplace, the article went on to report that Black women face a concrete ceiling, making career progression even more difficult. This isn't a secret in the Black community, and there are people with similar experiences in this country. There are some similarities between the lifestyle in the U.S.A. and the U.K. that Black women share, which may lend itself to the findings of these studies and may also contribute to how Black women in both countries experience menopause. A Trade Union Congress (TUC) report highlighted that almost one-third (31%) of Black and minority ethnic (BME) women reported 'being unfairly passed over for or denied a promotion at work' (TUC, 2020). It is worth referencing Vaina Lumbiwa's experience here and how she was turned down for a job in the U.K. because her natural hair was deemed 'inappropriate' (Ridley, 2023). This is not an isolated incident. 'Hair that is deemed as acceptable, professional and "corporate" the world over is often based on Western standards of straight, neat and obedient hair,' states Grace Mansah-Owusu, an organisational psychologist in Oxford, in her article on discrimination in the workplace (2023). The villainisation of Black women's hair continues to this day.

Now, you may be wondering about the relevance of this information to the menopause, but consider the impact of being pressured to change your appearance to fit in or be accepted by your peers or employer. How might that impact your self-worth at the realisation that your natural look has been deemed not good enough and, therefore, unacceptable? According to one study in this country, 'one in five Black women feel societal pressured to straighten their hair for work' (Eneje, 2021). Women resort to straightening their hair using relaxer kits that contain chemicals like phthalates and parabens. These ingredients are endocrine disruptors which intensify menopause symptoms, primarily hormones that regulate your mood, appetite and cognitive function relating to concentration and memory. Furthermore, these ingredients may increase the risk of uterine cancer (Bellamy, 2023). The World Afro Day campaign call for the Equality Act to protect against afro hair discrimination in the U.K. is a positive step in the right direction, but it doesn't stop there, (Mohdin, 2024). There is another possibility that might give rise to challenges when it comes to Black women's experience of the menopause. That is the 'strong Black' Woman' archetype, which describes Black women as being resilient and self-sufficient.

What does this have to do with the menopause, you ask?

This phenomenon of the Strong Black Woman is 'characterized as emotionally restrained, hyper-independent, nurturing and resilient, and she is not fazed by anything or anyone' (Dei, 2022). These are admirable qualities, as I'm sure you will agree. In fact, my friends and I advocate for these qualities and suppress any emotions or behaviours contrary to the ideal strong Black woman. This is how the circle of women around me behaved, and was advised that I, too, should be 'strong'. I later learnt that being this way could protect me from life's challenges as I got older, and behaving in any other way was frowned upon. It was not until recently that I learnt that this was a stereotype derived from the 'mammy caricature' during slavery. If you haven't looked into this phenomenon, I encourage you to do so to understand more about it. Regardless, being strong and resilient in the face of adversity are admirable qualities, and on the surface, I see no issue presenting myself this way. After all, we all want to be strong and have it together, and women are generally valued when they show up this way. Being an emotionally strong woman is the goal of every woman, states Mitzi Bockmann (2021), a life and love coach, in her article on the Thrive website. However, constantly showing up in this way can come across as being capable of withstanding life's challenges without needing support and that you are pretty much able to do practically everything yourself, like a super woman. On the face of it, you will appear to others as if you have your life all together, which, again, is admirable, but is that really a true picture?

Black women are generally seen as being emotionally guarded, hiding their hurts and struggles to live up to the stereotype of being self-sacrificing and self-sufficient, wearing a mask and groaning under 'weight' of this the burden. Psychologists will tell you that buried or repressed emotions seek expression in other ways; these are soul wounds that show up as chronic sicknesses in later years (hypertension and anxiety were two expressions of my soul wounds). This might be why Black women have the most long-term health conditions of any other ethnic group, according to a study carried out by King's College London (Soley-Bori, 2023). The most common conditions experienced are chronic pain, asthma, hypertension, anxiety and depression. Women are already particularly vulnerable to depression in menopause due to the drop in progesterone levels, which affects the way you respond to stress both physically and emotionally. Having to live up to a social ideal can only add to your stress levels. Freud, one of the fathers of psychology, discovered links between repression of emotion and physical symptoms nearly a century ago, and there has been a plethora of research since, about the link between repressed emotions manifesting in the physical in the form of sickness. The increased rate of hypertension in Black women might not only be the result of cumulative stress, but the ingredients used in the food they eat and cooking methods, more on diet in the next section of this chapter.

Living up to the 'strong Black woman' ideal is unrealistic, in my view, as it encourages women to suppress their emotions and deny the essence of who they are by showing up as society and culture dictate. Add in racism and discrimination, and you have a recipe for more stress in life. Attempting to live this way for many years, particularly in my teens and early adult years, made for a difficult life. I rarely asked for help, thinking that I needed to be confident and self-sufficient or I would be viewed as a failure in my community. I refused to show any emotions that might be considered weak and stuffed down my hurt and tears as if I were invincible, not realising they would come up and be expressed in my later years. Having come into this awareness, I am of the view that trying to live up to what I can only describe as an unachievable ideal and the stress of policing my behaviour and emotions contributed in some way to the health challenges I've experienced over the years. Sadly, the extent of carrying a high stress load has far wider health implications for Black women. High stress levels can cause sleep disruptions, which Black women experience at a higher rate, as well as hormone imbalance, appetite and temperature dysregulation (Michigan News, 2022). You might recall that hot flashes and night sweats are symptoms experienced more severely in menopausal Black women. Increased rates of obesity, hypertension, vertigo and high cholesterol, symptomatic of metabolic syndrome, are experienced in high rates in Black communities, too (Gaillard, 2018). Reducing stress has to be a priority at any given time and even more so in menopause, as we have less of our precious hormones to help us deal with life's challenges. The 'strong Black woman' phenomenon is a huge subject to tackle, and it deserves more attention than I can give it here.

Upon reflection, it would be of great benefit to women in the U.K if studies similar to the SWAN and Fawcett and Runnymede Trust studies were carried out, as it would provide a rich pool of knowledge to fully understand the extent of the impact on Black women's overall health during menopause and even on other women from marginalised backgrounds. Challenging structural racism is an ongoing battle, and reporting experiences will encourage policymakers to keep racism on the table when shaping or amending existing policies. Showing up as your authentic self is also important. Society will not be challenged if women give in to the pressure not to look like their natural selves for fear of being overlooked for certain jobs or promotions at work or not being generally accepted. Furthermore, how will the way women are treated and viewed ever shift if discrimination and cultural expectations are not challenged? There is a lot to unpack when trying to understand Black women's experiences, and these studies shed some light on why this may be the case.

Another factor to consider is surgical menopause, caused by medication or surgery, such as hysterectomy, whereby the uterus and ovaries are removed. According to gynaecologic oncologist Kemi Doll of the University of Washington, having a hysterectomy due to uterine fibroids contributes to early menopause in Black women (Rabin, 2022) I talk about my experience of having fibroids in Chapter 3. After being assessed by a naturopathic consultant, I learnt that my diet and lifestyle had caused estrogen dominance, which contributed to the growth of fibroids that caused me years of misery. The only option offered to me when I was first referred to the gynaecologist was a hysterectomy, and I had to fight to have a less invasive procedure. Changing my diet and using natural products did, however, help with symptoms and stopping their growth. Having fibroids was a teachable experience, as I learnt so much about what and how we eat and the impact of food on our physical and emotional well-being. It's shocking that some Black women in the '80s and '90s were denied less-invasive treatments for fibroids and only offered hysterectomies, hurling them into early menopause and denying them the opportunity to have children. Today, due to the awareness of other procedures, more women are demanding less-invasive and alternative treatments for fibroids, even if they don't want to start a family. It's worth mentioning here that on rare occasions, fibroids can return post menopause, but the reason for this occurring is unknown. I await in anticipation for explanations as to why this is the case, as I am currently supporting a client with post-menopausal fibroids.

It would be remiss of me if I did not mention other reasons early menopause can occur in Black women. Diet and lifestyle are two that require further exploration as to how they might have an impact on the menopausal experience. Caribbean foods have been described as flavoursome or, as one of my friends describes it, 'lip-smackin' food'. This is because the seasoning used in Caribbean cuisine can transform a bland dish into something that tastes magical. Jerk seasoning for example, is one of the many flavourings used to enhance the taste of Caribbean meals and is a cheaper option to buying fresh produce as it has a longer shelf life. The spicy flavour add a fiery kick to each dish, making meals irresistible. However, some seasonings are considered neurotoxins. Seasoning containing preservatives, such as monosodium glutamate (MSG), over-stimulate nerve cells and may cause headaches, palpitations, atopic dermatitis (a common form of eczema), asthma and hot flashes in women who are sensitive to MSG, according to a 2019 review in Comprehensive Reviews in Food Science and Food Safety (Horton & Myers, 2025). Given that these seasonings are used to marinate your meals, try replacing some seasonings with fresh produce, herbs and spices, like coriander, turmeric, chillies, garlic, onion, pimento and thyme, that will make your meals just as flavoursome and likely help your menopausal symptoms, too. Consider turmeric: it is an anti-inflammatory and can help reduce inflammation, joint pain and hot flashes. Pimento is often used to add flavour to soups or rice, and peas, helps balance estrogen. Eating onions every day is good for bone health. Why not try out some new ingredients to add tantalising flavours to your meals? There are so many different fresh ingredients available, so you don't have to stick to what you have used for many years.

How you cook your food is equally important when going through this transition. You may not know this, but a lot of Caribbean dishes are fried, and although cooking this way adds flavour to your food, eating fried food every day is likely to have an impact on your heart health and create inflammation in the body. This is important as the reduction of progesterone, our anti-inflammatory hormone during menopause, makes it more difficult for your body to manage inflammation. If you experience joint pain or gain weight, you may have a lot of inflammation in your body. Many degenerative diseases we see as a 'normal' part of ageing are triggered by chronic inflammation. Foods containing omega-3 fatty acids, such as flaxseed and oily fish, might help reduce joint pain and other inflammatory conditions. After all, prevention is better than a cure. A study carried out on 'women over 50 years old found that overindulging in fried foods can increase a person's risk of death, (Sun et al, 2019). Protein and fat-rich foods that have been heated to high temperatures to enhance flavour, colour and aroma can not only affect your hormones but can also shorten your life. Therefore, it is important to change how you cook at this stage of your life. If you have always eaten this way, you may have a fair amount of toxins and metabolic waste stored in your body, which can increase your risk of insulin resistance and hypertension.

There's a lot of research about how cooking food destroys some of its nutritional content, particularly in vegetables. I often advocate that my clients have at least one raw meal a day. A large salad is packed with nutrients and is naturally low in sodium and calories. Having fresh green juice every day can reduce the oxidated stress load in your body. Oxidated stress is not only caused by diet and what you put on your skin but lowered estrogen levels increase oxidated stress, too. Oxidated stress is ageing, causing fatigue, brain fog and greying hair. By changing your diet, you can slow the ageing process and improve symptoms of the menopause. Menopause is more than a physiological change, we have also established that it has psychosocial components. The environmental, social and emotional factors also influence a woman's response to this transition, which is why a holistic approach is necessary to support women on their menopause journey.

There is so much to consider when it comes to Black women's experience of the menopause, and I hope the information contained in this chapter gives you some concepts to consider as well as generate conversations with your peers about the issue. Most of this research was carried out in America; therefore, conducting studies in this country would be helpful for women to understand their menopause journey better. I don't make the assumption that discrimination and cultural expectations impact all Black women, and I am not of the view that these studies allude to that. Their findings give us a framework for understanding Black women's experiences of the menopause. I have a few friends who seem to be going through this transition with minimal symptoms, but the majority are struggling. If what you have read so far piques your interest, read studies that have been carried out on the subject and participate in research when the opportunity presents itself. This is how we ensure the needs of Black women and other marginalised groups are understood and catered to by medical professionals and policymakers.

Going through menopause presents women with physiological and psychological challenges which call for self-compassion and 'soft living'. I encourage you to seek a more simplified life, unburdened by stress wherever possible, one in which you are the priority, and you nurture your soul. Use the menopause as a time of reflection and carry out a life audit. This exercise really helped to shine the spotlight on all areas of my life and prioritise what should be more important to me at this stage of life. It also helped me start peeling back the layers of the persona I hid behind for so many years; I no longer feel the need to mask my vulnerabilities or live up to the ideals or stereotypes society buys into. It is not the end, as some people would like you to think, it can be a new beginning, a time to birth something new and meaningful. If you struggle with symptoms, seek advice and explore natural alternatives to manage symptoms, such as herbs and nutrition, that can alleviate symptoms. I discuss this in later chapters.

CHAPTER 6

How to Thrive Amidst Hormonal Changes

Hormones affect virtually every organ in our bodies; therefore, when we go through the change, we should not be too surprised to experience some unusual symptoms like tinnitus, dizziness, tingling or numbing sensations in the mouth, cold flushes, and even anxiety and depression. The emotional side of menopause isn't widely spoken about as we often frame menopause in terms of physical symptoms, and feelings of sadness, anxiety, loss of confidence and being overwhelmed are often missed. It is, therefore, important for us to pay attention to the emotional side of the menopause as psychological symptoms can be just as debilitating as physical symptoms. A lot of women I speak to struggle to cope with this change emotionally and feel kind of out of sorts. A few disclosed having negative thoughts towards the menopause and even anger. They felt that menopause was an attack on their womanhood, and they no longer felt sexy or productive. Their sex lives were practically non-existent and they didn't quite like how their bodies were changing or how they felt. Some women felt grief at no longer being able to conceive, even if they did not want to have any more children. Others were beset with anger, guilt and loneliness as they felt their youth slipping away, and they grieved the passage of time. Women are often faced with a change of identity, a new reality that opens them up to uncertainty about ageing.

Menopause throws up some uncomfortable questions for women, and we are still learning about the change because it has been shrouded in secrecy and as a taboo for so long. Women have, for the most part, had to try to figure things out for themselves and suffer in silence because of the stigma and myths surrounding the change. I had many questions going into perimenopause and questioned my mental health on some days because I occasionally felt unhinged. I lost confidence in my ability to learn new things; information just wouldn't stick, and I was forgetful. When speaking to a few friends of a similar age, I found that they, too, had similar experiences. A few had even lost confidence in driving, although they had been driving for many years. I felt unattractive as I struggled to shift stubborn fat and experienced skin flair ups on and off that went on for years. Having spoken to a few professionals who have worked with women going through hormonal changes and having studied hormones myself, it wasn't long before I was able to connect the dots, alleviating my fears.

I don't recall my mother ever going through menopause. She always appeared calm and was never one to complain about anything, so she either had very few symptoms or went down the natural route to treat her symptoms. I do recall her asking her friends to bring back dandelion herbs when they went to Jamaica on holiday. Dandelion herbs has amazing benefits for hormonal changes and is great for cleansing your liver. More information on herbs and supplements in later chapters.

It took me a while to come to terms with being in menopause, but once I accepted that it had arrived, I decided I would learn as much about it as I could to improve my health and vitality. Despite my new-found knowledge, I wasn't prepared for the emotions that came with this transition, like feelings of gloom, unworthiness and anxiety. I felt as if I had missed out on so much in life. Time, all of a sudden, became precious. I decided it was time for introspection, so I went to task, armed with my journal and pen and assessed everything and everyone, which relationships were adding value to my life and worth investing in, outdated beliefs, finances, career. I was doing a total life audit. I wanted a life that was meaningful and purposeful, but despite my eagerness to revamp things, my self-esteem was at rock bottom because of the symptoms I struggled with, like intrusive and negative thoughts. I unnecessarily criticised and berated myself for making even the smallest mistakes, along with my past failings. Without my precious hormones, I lost my self-compassion and was quite harsh on myself. It took a lot of inner healing to work through these emotions and start valuing myself again. You might recall how, in an earlier chapter, I said that repressed emotions would likely come up for expression at this time. Mine manifested as self-criticism along with health problems like hypertension.

What mostly stood out for me was the feeling of not being needed anymore. My children had grown up and had lives of their own. I was miserable in my career and desperately wanted more. I felt like I was being kicked out of life, and no one understood me. It didn't help that I had applied for a senior post and was rejected for a younger applicant. I started to grieve the life I once had. Resentment kicked in, and I found myself secretly envious of women who still had their families around them and who were thriving in their careers. Emotionally, I felt like I was drowning. I was unaware of the impact of low progesterone and estrogen on regulating my emotions, memory and decision making or how these hormones directly affected other hormones, like oxytocin and serotonin. My love hormone and feel-good hormone were depleting, and I realised that I was isolating myself and had fallen out of love with my then partner. Did you know that divorce rates are higher in midlife? The loss of attraction to your partner and losing interest in intimacy are some of the reasons given for divorce. This was my experience, and it seems to be the experience of many women who decide to walk away from their relationships.

Some women who approached their doctors for support were told to accept the natural process, without appreciating the importance of intimacy in relationships, and the fear and anxiety some women may experience in that area, particularly if their relationships are suffering or they no longer feel like themselves. The response of some medical professionals towards women going through the menopause is disconcerting as women are left feeling ignored, undermined and undervalued when speaking about intimacy. I recently learnt on the menopause practitioner course I completed, that doctors and gynaecologists have very little training in perimenopause and menopause and are, therefore, unclear as to how women should manage symptoms (Richardson et al.2023). Consequently, women are left to seek alternative treatments or suffer in silence, according to Susan Dominus in her article 'Women have been misled about menopause,' published in the *New York Times* (2023). It's as if women are expected to give up intimacy now that they are in menopause. They should just suck it up and get on with life when men are readily prescribed Viagra if they struggle with intimacy. This typifies gender ageism. If you are worried about intimacy, find a health coach who specialises in menopause. There are also natural products and foods that can help with your hormones. You will be amazed at how changing your diet can help eliminate some menopause symptoms. Dark chocolate, oats and pineapple, for example, increase serotonin production and improve your mood. If you experience low libido, try red clover herb, which is really beneficial for boosting your libido. Speak to your health practitioner if you are taking medication, as some herbs may reduce the effectiveness of your medication.

Having a conversation with your partner about how you are feeling and also about the physical changes that come with menopause is important to prevent misunderstanding. Don't shut your partner out. There is a lot of educational material online you can share with them. Also, be aware that your partner may be going through a change, too, as some men experience andropause, recently termed 'manopuase' in midlife, with symptoms similar to the menopause. I cover andropause in Chapter 4. Andropause isn't widely spoken about, even though there can be health risks. Go back to that chapter, and if you recognise signs of andropause in your partner encourage him to seek advice as this will avoid putting a strain on your relationship and help improve both of your transitions through these changes.

In my quest to improve my low mood and the emotions that kept me feeling less than, I had to face some truths. I was growing weary of being miserable on the inside and wearing a mask of happiness and contentment on the outside. It was time for me to take control, rip off the mask and bare my soul. It was time for soul-care. I spent hours daily, pouring over books and research materials. I attended many courses on personal development and healing. Getting a life coach was the best thing I did for my healing, as my coach was amazing at getting me to take responsibility for my life. She held up a mirror to my life, which helped me acknowledge areas where self-doubt was holding me back and how, unconsciously, I had been limiting myself. Coupled with my knowledge of using nutrition to manage hormones, I decided it was time to write a new story. Menopause would be my new beginning. What I've learnt will, hopefully, give you some clarity and peace of mind as it did me.

So, here goes…

By the time you enter the menopause, you are likely to have spent most of your life playing different role, being a parent, wife, aunt, grandmother, friend and student, and may have worn many professional hats. As you approach this transition, the realisation that you are nearing retirement can be scary. After all, for most of us, our jobs give us a sense of identity and belonging. If someone asked me who I am, I would introduce myself by my name and my occupation. I was my job, and, I guess, that is how society tell us to define ourselves. So, now that I am in menopause, which occurs at a time not too far off from retirement, I have some anxiety about the future. I describe the menopause as a period of shifting sands. This transition creates instability and, to some extent, an identity crisis. It is a new reality that brings uncertainty for some women. Throw in symptoms of the menopause like hot flushes, disrupted sleep, aches and pains, fatigue and irritability, and anyone would be hard-pressed to feel confident. You might find that you feel uncharacteristically depressed. Even more so when you reflect over the years and come to the realisation that you put your life on hold to attend to the needs of others and became comfortable putting your needs last. One lady I coached described this as a woman's needs unacknowledged.

Menopause is a way of waking you up to your needs, which, for the most part, have been last on your to-do list. It's a time when your soul cries out for expression as you realise the clock is ticking, retirement is no longer in the distant future, and all the things you've wanted to achieve, like passions unfulfilled, are now threatened with never being birthed. It was when I realised that my life was not as meaningful and fulfilling as I thought it was. I bought into what society told me happiness and fulfilment were and sought happiness externally instead of connecting to my soul. For some women, this is when feelings of resentment, anger, worry and sadness rise to the surface as they neglected the essence of who they are and lived a life dictated by societal and cultural norms. This was the primary reason I expanded my coaching practice to include helping menopausal women connect to the essence of who they truly are so they can unlock a new level of confidence, joy and vitality. Prioritising yourself is important if you want to make the most of your menopausal years and beyond. You may recall, in chapter 3, that when you repress your true self and emotions by censoring yourself and policing your thoughts, unresolved emotions and conversations left unsaid get absorbed into the body, which can make menopause a more uncomfortable experience.

How is this so?

We deposit unresolved emotions throughout our bodies that we can recall at any given moment, similar to how the brain stores memories. Left unexpressed, these emotions may cause tension in the body, triggering disease and causing limiting beliefs like self-doubt, self-loathing and low self-esteem. Adverse childhood experiences and trying to live up to societal standards are often the root causes of these emotions as is how you perceive your place in the world. Throw in symptoms of perimenopause and subsequently menopause, and you might find your confidence level plummet and experience waves of anxiety and depression. Both estrogen and progesterone affect your mood, controlling the production of 'feel good' endorphins, and when levels fluctuate, you are left with less of these hormones to deal with daily challenges or achieve a state of homeostasis. This is often when unresolved emotions surface in unhealthy ways. Not all women experience bouts of anxiety or depression; some experience irritability, low tolerance levels and even angry outbursts. Talking through your emotions is important for your emotional and physical health.

When I studied reflexology, I learnt about Chinese philosophies on how emotions affect specific organs of the body (Chinese

Medicine Living, 2012), which makes for interesting reading, to say the least. They found that the heart is the source of joy and is very sensitive to emotional states. Feelings of guilt, remorse and deceit can weaken the heart, causing symptoms such as a lack of enthusiasm, mental restlessness, anxiety and depression. On a physiological level, we might experience insomnia, heart palpitations, poor memory and a lack of concentration. The lungs can be affected by grief, excessive pensiveness, feelings of invalidation, being overshadowed, smothering and sadness. These emotions can trigger physiological symptoms such as asthma, frequent colds and other respiratory problems. Feelings of anger, irritability, frustration, resentment, jealousy and envy can affect the liver, causing headaches, premenstrual stress and muscular tension (Vanbuskirk, 2024).

Hormonal imbalance will likely intensify these emotions and, in turn, jeopardise your health. Going through this transition is like being on a rollercoaster, and if the emotional and cognitive symptoms of menopause are ignored, can develop into depression. Don't ignore how you feel. Get support from a trusted friend or health coach. There is no shame in seeking help. If you are worried about your confidence and self-esteem, give yourself the space you need to understand and accept the changes you're experiencing, however long that takes. Acknowledge and connect with the emotions that might have limited you for many years. A good coach will help to release you from the cage of limiting beliefs and help you navigate your menopause journey. Don't buy into the myth that menopause is the end; it's a transition that requires guidance, acceptance, understanding and information to get you into a space of renewal and growth. Prioritising yourself is important at this time, and there are resources available to you. I am both impressed and excited to witness the growth of menopause support groups around the country as they offer women a safe space to give and receive support. Look online for groups you can attend. There are some virtual groups, too. Whatever you decide, don't suffer in silence. Reach out for support.

Hormone Replacement Therapy (HRT) is an option for mood swings, but not every woman chooses this option primarily because of the health risks. I encourage you to speak to your health provider for current information on HRT as treatments advance over the years. Managing symptoms does not need to cost the earth, nor do you need to take drastic action. I mention below some steps you can take to help you feel better about yourself and your menopause journey.

We hear so much about gratitude. Every guru worth their salt will tell you how important it is to be grateful. Granted, when symptoms like hot flashes, irritability, headaches and brain fog intensify, being thankful is not likely high on your agenda. However, focusing on positive emotions, such as gratitude, reduces stress hormones like cortisol and promotes a sense of wellbeing. Cortisol is not bad, 'we need cortisol to kick-start us in the morning, it's what motivates us, allowing us the energy to get out of bed' (Positive Pause, 2020). But when levels are too high for too long, it can cause adrenal fatigue, which means there will be less estrogen in our bodies to help us manage stress. Being grateful makes life feel that much better. It stops you from spiralling into negativity, which robs you of your inner peace and happiness. According to science, including gratitude practices in your routine, like keeping a gratitude journal, can increase your wellbeing, happiness and overall mood. Having less estrogen and progesterone reduces serotonin levels, which is likely to trigger feeling overwhelmed, sadness and anxiety. Taking a supplement like valerian root will not only help with hot flashes but also help you get a better night's sleep, improving your mood. Other supplements that can help with your low mood are evening primrose and St John's Wort.

You have heard the saying, 'Your thoughts create your reality?' It reminds me of the Bible verse in Proverbs, chapter 23, verse 7: 'For as he thinketh in his heart, so is he.' There is so much truth to this. Your thoughts really do influence your emotions, which determine the actions you are likely to take. For example, if you equate menopause with becoming unattractive or falling apart, you will continually criticise and judge yourself. These messages will be reflected in your body, and you will appear to others as being lacklustre and depressed. You will look unhappy, and your shoulders will be slumped and rounded. Therefore, it is important to feed your mind properly. Plant seeds you want to grow and harvest in the future. Spend time each day in silent contemplation. Listen to the messages you tell yourself. Are they positive? Are they filled with love and compassion, or are they unsupportive, like regret, resentment and sorrow? In Shakespeare's famous play, Hamlet tells Rosencrantz, 'There is nothing either good or bad, but thinking makes it so.' Given this statement, it is important that you feed your mind with positive affirmations to challenge negative or unhelpful thoughts.

Regular prayer has benefits similar to meditation in reducing anxiety and stress and evoking inner peace. We need peace in our lives as the menopause hurls us into a period of intense symptoms. People tend to think of prayer as being primarily for religious people, but there are many people who are not religious who pray. Many people look to a higher power for comfort. I recall reading an article shortly after lockdown that reported Google searches for prayer skyrocketed in March 2020 (Bentzen, 2021). For me, knowing that there is a higher power out there who I view as God, gave me hope, a sense of security and helped me value myself even more during the transition, especially when I had occasional bouts of feeling overwhelmed. Prayer is a part of soul care.

Working on yourself, on your mindset, and accepting where you are in life are important for a better menopause experience. Accepting yourself for who you are is equally important. The bottom line is that you are the only person who can change how you feel. Some people think that changing their physical circumstances, such as moving to a new city or town or changing employment, can improve their emotions, and it may initially work, but it is likely only temporary. Wherever you go, you carry your emotions with you. You cannot escape them. This is the time to really get to know yourself and connect with your soul before making any decisions about your physical circumstances. What is also important is taking the time to pause and really listen to your soul. What does it say? What do you need at this time? We are not taught to really listen to our souls because, as a society, we've shut down our ability to hear our inner voices. We become proficient at achieving things, but it comes at a cost: the silencing of our internal voices. Furthermore, we listen to gurus, religious leaders and politicians to tell us how to live to the exclusion of our souls. It is time to resolve in your heart not to allow other people's opinions of you to have an impact on the way you live your life. Trying to live up to other people's ideals or philosophies can be catastrophic for your emotional wellbeing. Don't allow society to dictate how you should live your life.

Spend some time reassessing your life. Are you doing what you love? If not, why not? Do you have a passion you abandoned due to other commitments? Revisit it now that you have more time on your hands. If your circumstances does not permit you to make major changes, set some goals and implement small changes until you can achieve them. This could also be the time to find a new role that will satisfy you, like volunteering or enrolling on a course. Doing so will also help improve your self-esteem and mood. Find a reason to enjoy life. Immerse yourself in positive pursuits that allow you to grow. Expand your social or spiritual life to replace inward, self-critical patterns.

Although challenging your mindset is super important in menopause, watching your diet is just as important. There are great foods you can incorporate in your diet to improve your mood . I call them mood boosting foods like oily fish, which is a great source of omega-3 fatty acids that might help regulate your mood. Bananas are always in season, they contain magnesium and potassium, helping improve your sleep as well as your energy levels. Plantains have similar properties to help improve your mood and are a daily staple in Costa Rica, which is probably why it is called the 'happy country'. I like to add sea moss to my smoothie, a great source of folic acid that boosts serotonin levels, your happy hormone. I cover more healthy nutritional information in the next chapter.

Diet and exercise go together like peas in a pod. Rarely do we see dietary advice without mentioning the added benefits of exercise, which makes sense, given the lifestyle changes we want to make during this transition. Exercise boosts your body image and health, and with less estrogen and testosterone, weight-bearing exercise becomes even more crucial for preserving muscle mass and reducing the risk of osteoporosis. Exercise might also reduce hot flashes and help with your mood, according to a study on the impact of high-load resistance training on bone mineral density in osteoporosis and osteopenia (Kitsuda et al., 2021). Another great form of exercise is dancing. I love to dance. It's a wonderful form of self-expression and an equally great way to release stuck emotions by increasing serotonin levels. So, put on some music and start swinging and gyrating those hips. It's a great way to lose weight and boost your health. Have you ever tried belly dancing? This is another favourite of mine that is great for keeping your hips flexible. Belly dancing is also great for pelvic health, which, in turn, can help with urine incontinence, another symptom of low estrogen. If you don't feel brave enough to join a class, head over to YouTube where you will find many tutorials.

Getting physical is great, but so is rest, and getting a good night's sleep is perfect for reducing cortisol levels, as well as allowing your cells to repair. Practicing good sleep hygiene, like having a bedtime routine, will help sync your body clock. Avoid stimulants like alcohol and caffeine. Also, reduce screen time in the evening and turn off devices at least an hour before you go to bed so as not to disrupt melatonin production, which will help you get a good night's sleep. Taking care of your soul is important when going through the menopause and is one of the reasons I encourage my clients to focus on soul care. Incorporating these practices into your lifestyle is a great start to feeling better about yourself and improving your emotional wellbeing throughout your menopause journey.

CHAPTER 7

The Hidden Dangers of Poor Nutrition

You are hungry, so you eat. Most of our relationship with food is primarily to alleviate hunger and provide our bodies with the required nutrients to keep us fit and healthy. Since our bodies are in a constant state of renewal, they draw on the food we consume to build new cells. The food we eat gives our bodies the information and materials required to function at optimum levels. It makes sense, then, that what we eat is vital to create healthy cells, healthy systems and, in turn, healthy bodies.

How does this relate to the menopause and the andropause?

As you read on, you will learn about the link between food and this transition and how you can make it a smoother, less worrisome experience. But first, let's look at the importance of nutrition.

When we experience illness or feel generally unwell, we often go to our doctors to get a check-up. Some of us will probably nip to our local health store or pharmacy to purchase supplements, but what about our dietary habits? Neglecting to provide your body with sufficient nutrients is usually the root cause of sickness. Nutrition is the foundation for health and development, and there are a few fundamentals to consider when planning to eat healthier.

I would encourage the following to optimise your health as you go through 'The Change.'

- Include small amounts of protein with every meal. Proteins are your muscles' building blocks and protein becomes even more crucial as you go through the menopause because of the danger of sarcopenia.

- Consume fruit and vegetables daily. They are rich in phytochemical and antioxidants that strengthen the immune system and help your body get rid of oxidated stress, which can make hot flashes and night sweats worse.

- Eat grass-fed meat as it is higher in antioxidants and omega-3 fatty acids than meat from animals raised on grain

- Limit your consumption of ultra processed foods because some contain high levels of sugar which can raise blood sugar levels, putting you in danger of insulin resistance

- It's important to stay hydrated because hot flashes and night sweats can cause significant fluid loss. Sip water often throughout the day.

- Listen to your body.

These fundamentals essentially constitute a diet that will optimise your health and keep you alive longer. Consider what you have eaten today or even this week, were most of the meals you consumed nutritious?

You may agree that these fundamentals are easy enough to incorporate into your everyday life, but is this the case? Unfortunately, not for many. This is primarily because our lifestyles have become more hectic, limiting the time we have to prepare wholesome meals. There aren't enough hours in the day, is a common lament, especially if you are in full time employment, self-employed or enrolled in full-time education. Eating on the go, which, for many, includes large amounts of ultra processed foods, has become the norm. These foods can wreak havoc on our health and make some symptoms like hot flashes and palpitations worse.

Let's take a look at processed foods more closely.

Processed food is any food that has 'been altered in some way during preparation, whether by freezing, canning, baking or drying' (Champion, 2021). This process provides products with a longer shelf-life, stabilises animal products and removes harmful bacteria.

Some processed food, those that are ultra processed, like cereal bars and ready meals contain an unhealthy amount of salt, sugar and fat, all in an attempt to improve the flavour after the food has been altered and adulterated. The large consumption of these foods is responsible for increasing levels of obesity, heart disease and diabetes according to the National Health Service.

But not all 'processed' foods are bad for you. For example, oil is pressed from olives to make olive oil. This involves a process, but the end product is not bad. Naturally fermented foods, such as Kimchi, sauerkraut, Kombucha and yoghurt made from raw, pastured cow's milk, have gone through a natural fermentation process and are very good for your body, even though they have all undergone a process that technically makes them processed foods (Rosenbloom, 2017).

Reading labels on products has never been more crucial than it is today. What is more shocking to me is that ultra processed foods can be addictive because they work on our bodies in ways similar to addictive hard drugs. They are absorbed into the bloodstream quickly and in high doses and can actually give us a 'rush' or a 'high' similar to hard drugs as they stimulate the reward system of the brain that drives our behaviour towards pleasurable stimuli and away from painful ones. Foods such as chocolate, pizza, crisps, cakes and ice cream are considered pleasure foods for many because they release dopamine, or that feel-good factor, the same way drugs and alcohol do (Gearhardt et al., 2023). Sweet and flavours are considered to be as addictive. Consider the rich savouriness of soya sauce, parmesan cheese, aged meat and even Chinese food. These all use a flavour enhancer called Monosodium Glutamate (MSG), which is a naturally occurring amino acid in some meat, dairy and vegetables (Warner, 2024). You may have read about or heard about MSG a while back when there was a lot of media attention on the dangers of consuming it because it may be harmful to the body.

According to Dr Lundell Dwight, a world-renowned heart surgeon, processed foods can destroy the walls of our blood vessels by causing chronic inflammation, resulting in cholesterol sticking to the walls, leading to plaque and, in turn, heart disease (American Academy, 2019). Having this knowledge made me question how I was eating even more and whether processed food had any benefits at all. Whilst I do not disapprove of all processed foods, as some processed foods like frozen fruit and vegetables, as well as canned fish have nutritional benefits; I think it important to consider how the food you are eating is processed and, most importantly, what has been added. This is crucial as we age as we want to reduce the risk of causing ourselves ill health. I will touch on this more in subsequent chapters.

The influx of low-fat meals in our supermarkets and weight loss programmes popping up everywhere is the food industry's response to these epidemics, heart disease and obesity. However, the process used to lower the fat in our foods, hydrogenation, involves altering the structure of vegetable oils to replace solid fats, which can cause high cholesterol (Mayo Clinic, 2025). That's pretty scary, to say the least, and there's more. Many low-fat foods contain high levels of sugar to improve the taste and texture once provided by the naturally occurring fat. Consequently, they can contain as many calories as their full fat equivalent (Nguyen et al. 2016). The human brain is nearly 60% fat (Northwestern Medicine, 2024), so please do not eliminate healthy fats from your diet, as they play a vital role in every bodily function. For those of you who, like me, struggle to bring discipline to their eating habits, there is a healthy way to shed those pounds. Leading experts are calling for slimmers to adopt the lesser known Victorian diet, eating like our 19th century forebears who ate a vegetable-rich diet.

The mid-Victorian era, between the years of 1850 and 1872, was a 'mini golden age of nutrition', according to Dr Judith Rowbotham, of the University of Plymouth, who co-authored research with Dr Paul Clayton, of the Institute of Food, Brain and Behaviour. (Davies, 2015). Mid-Victorians lived without modern diagnostics, drugs, surgery or contraception. Despite that, and because of the high nutrient density of their diets, their lifespan was as long as ours and their health was likely significantly better (Davies, 2015).

As dairy and meat became staples following the shift in Britain's agricultural policy, milk came to be viewed as being extremely important to the health and wellbeing of the nation and is still advocated as such by professionals today. I still have fond memories of my youth when our friendly milkman delivered milk to our door from a local farm. I rushed to the door to bring in the milk and sat patiently at the table, excited as my mother poured the creamy substance over my cereal. We were also given milk daily at school to ensure we received the recommended daily allowance of calcium as a provision of the Free Milk Act 1946, but is dairy still healthy for us to consume today?

Let's look more closely at today's milk.

Way back when milk came from cows that were grass-fed. They roamed outside all day, grazing on grass, which meant our milk contained larger amounts of fatty acids and omega-3 fat, as well as Vitamin A and other nutrients inherent in grass and weeds. The soil was rich in nutrients that fed the grass, which fed the cows. Nutrients that reduce inflammation in the body were passed on to the people consuming dairy products), providing greater protection, (Alothman et al., 2019). Due to increasing demand for meat and dairy, there has been an alarming move towards intensive farming, resulting in dairy cows being packed in sheds and fed genetically modified protein, drugs and hormones in order to boost production and growth (Animal Welfare Institute, n.d.). You may not be aware, but hormones cannot be 'cooked out' and are therefore ingested by anyone who eats non-organic meats or dairy products, increasing the amount of hormones in their systems.

These findings were both alarming and disconcerting, to say the least, and I found myself pondering even more to the point where I obsessed about my health and diet, and I wanted to find out how I should be eating for The Change.

CHAPTER 8

Nourishing Through the Change

THe standard Western diet can be characterised as being high in animal products, modern wheat products, processed foods and sodas. It's low in vegetables, fermented foods and, to a lesser extent, fruit. Common ingredients found in the Western diet include high fructose corn syrup, trans fat or partially hydrogenated oils, sugar, bleached and enriched flours, artificial flavours and many other chemical additives that strip food of all or most of its nutritional value. (Clemente-Suárez, 2023). An increase in hypertension, heart disease, diabetes and obesity has been linked to the Western diet and we have established that products from concentrated animal feeding operations (CAFO) and/or non-organic animal products likely contribute to the growth in hormonal imbalances. Consuming ultra processed food burden the body with additional stress and calories. This food is lower in nature's dazzling array of healing enzymes, vitamins and minerals (Clemente-Suárez, 2023). Therefore, it would be imprudent for us to think that what we eat does not have an effect on menopausal symptoms. Despite health professionals reporting the dangers of these foods, fast food restaurants are popping up everywhere and are often heaving with customers whilst, until recently, healthier cafes and restaurants were struggling to fill their seats. Things are starting to change, though, as the trend in plant-based foods gives rise to vegan and raw food restaurants, particularly in larger cities, and they compete pretty well with traditional cafes and restaurants.

According to the International Menopause Society (IMS) (2022, p. 1), women in midlife typically gain an average of 0.5 kg (about 1 lb) a year due to hormonal disruption that begins in the perimenopause years and continues throughout the menopause. I can definitely attest to the weight gain. Since going through this transition, I have gone up a dress size and a bit as my estrogen deficiency had pushed fatty deposits into my thighs and abdomen. The same occurs in men due to decreased testosterone. Eating a diet high in fat, sugar and processed foods not only increases your waist size but can lead to insulin resistance or sensitivity. Unbalanced insulin levels make it nearly impossible to manage your symptoms, particularly hot flashes and weight gain (Stills, 2013). Given these factors, it is easy to understand how we can struggle to manage our weight during this transition.

For some women, a recurring symptom is hormone-related headaches. The sudden drop of estrogen following a prolonged period of elevation can cause severe headaches once you enter the menopause. MacGregor (2009) puts this down to fluctuating hormone levels. Food rich in tyramine, such as pickles, alcohol, chocolates and cheese, should be avoided or reduced as they can trigger migraines in those sensitive to migraines (Metcalf, 2024). Spicy foods, a favourite of mine, can trigger hot flashes because the capsaicin in chillies and piperine in black pepper dilates blood vessels. If you're prone to flushing, overly dilated vessels tend to magnify this symptom and the sensation of heat you get from the spice will only make things worse (Collins, 2023). I now only have one or two spicy meals per week, which may be why I no longer get hot flashes.

In the previous chapter, I looked at practices in the food industry, such as the use of genetically modified feed for animals and hormones to speed up the growth process. The consequence of this is that we are being flooded with extra hormones that disrupt our own hormonal levels and have far-reaching effects on our bodies and minds, but how does food influence our minds and, in particular, our mood during the menopause?

In the 1970s, Dr Judith and Dr Richard Wurtman discovered that when we consumed carbohydrate dense foods such as potatoes, bread and pasta, serotonin is released which calms and relaxes (Wurtman & Frusztajer, 2009). Is this the reason carbohydrate-dense foods and foods rich in fat and sugar are often viewed as comfort foods, because they soothe us? Craving sweet foods during the premenstrual phase of the monthly cycle may be attributed to the calming effects of these foods. Similarly, during the menopause, we are likely to crave particular foods due to changes to the adrenal glands, making us more sensitive to stress hormones. Consequently, we are likely to suffer from anxiety and irritation, which can make some of us overeat, even more so if you are prone to comfort eating. Menopause symptoms, such as fatigue, depression and anxiety, may intensify food cravings. Overindulging in simple carbohydrates, fatty foods and alcohol increases serotonin, but not without consequences. As we have discovered, eating these foods can lead to unpleasant symptoms, including weight gain, a hyper stimulated nervous system, fatigue, depression and anxiety. Reducing these types of foods or completely cutting them out is the key to enjoying good health. Your body has the innate intelligence and capacity to heal and regenerate itself. It is self-healing and self-regulating if you give it the right foods. Begin by wiping the slate clean and getting back to simplicity in your diet.

Food should be healing and light to the body, particularly as we go through The Change. Scientists have proven that everything is energy or vibration, and everything vibrates at a different frequency: the air we breathe, our thoughts and our food. All food consumed either connects us to or disconnects us from nature. Food containing less energy or vibration will have an impact on the function of your cells. The lower the energy or frequency vibration a cell has, the closer it gets to destruction. Live foods vibrate at a much higher frequency than cooked foods. You may remember experiments with potatoes in science class that were able to run a clock or light up a small light bulb. This is the real energy that comes from food. It's not a myth. Foods that have a higher vibration include those rich in chlorophyll, such as leafy greens, spinach, kale, barley grass, wheat grass and algae. These foods also place less stress on the digestive system and are excellent for cleansing and oxygenating the blood, as well as boosting the immune system. I encourage you to fill your shopping basket with these foods as they will optimise your health as you adjust to this transition. I will discuss these foods, as well as others that are beneficial in later chapters. It is clear, then, that what we eat, as well as our mindset, determines how we experience the menopause to a large extent.

As a wellness practitioner specializing in menopause, I get asked a lot of questions about the best diet for the menopause and the andropause, primarily because conflicting advice abounds. Before embarking on this new career, I trawled the internet searching for a diet that would cure my ailments and menopausal symptoms. Some diets were somewhat extreme. They banned a lot of foods and beverages, such as alcohol and carbohydrates. I am not one for extreme diets and would not admonish my clients for eating particular foods or consuming alcohol. Everything in moderation is my motto, if you are relatively healthy. If your health is compromised in any way, that motto does not apply to you. I do have one rule: ensure that whatever food or drink you consume is of good quality, organic and natural, as these foods have more antioxidant compounds.

We have already established foods that we need to reduce in our diet to minimise symptoms and foods we should eat to increase vitality. Eating food in its natural state will benefit you immensely as you go through The Change. I do draw from a lot of the principles of a raw food diet; however, I do not advocate it as the only answer to improving one's health during The Change.

Many celebrities have adopted a raw, vegan lifestyle to increase their intake of essential vitamins, minerals and enzymes as well as lose weight and maintain or achieve a more youthful glow. It is also great for the environment since organic foods reduce the harmful chemicals used in agribusiness.

Megan Fox adopted a strict raw vegan diet for one year. Madonna previously adopted a regime of vegetables, fruit, grains, nuts and beans in place of meat, sugar and dairy. Demi Moore put her stunning looks down to Pilates and a raw vegan diet plan, and Sting has kept up a raw vegan regime for years. What is noticeable about most of these celebrities is that they're likely to be experiencing the menopause/andropause, and they look radiant and youthful. There is definitely something to be said about this diet. When we are going through the menopause or the andropause, we need to maintain a nutritious diet to reduce or eliminate symptoms. We have become accustomed to eating routinely, and for the most part, we pay minimal attention to what we are eating, especially when in a hurry or dealing with the demands of the day. What you may or may not know is that every bit of food we eat carries a vibration or frequency, as everything is made up of energy. Fresh fruit and vegetables from a plant, tree or vine carry a much higher vibration than any food that is processed, keeping our bodies light. Food containing a high nutritional value such as nuts, lacto-fermented vegetables and kefir, berries, wheatgrass, barley green, spirulina and blue and green algae energise and create homeostasis in the body. In fact, any food you consume in its pure, raw form as nature intended is infused with energy from the sun, and that energy causes it to vibrate at a high frequency that benefits both your physical and spiritual health, which is an indication that food does more than nourish you physically. Food also carries energy and vibration.

I recall when I changed my diet by cutting out fast foods, meat, ultra processed food, sodium and salt, I noticed that I had more energy and a positive mindset. I must note here that not all salt is bad for you; Himalayan salt contains over 80 minerals, which can help your body balance your pH levels, remove toxins and help absorb nutrients, unlike table salt, which is processed removing practically all minerals. Animals carry vibrations that can be transferred to humans when we consume their meat. An animal that has spent its life living in grueling circumstances is likely to be anxious and depressed, so when you eat meat from CAFOs, you can absorb the animal's negative energy. Animals that are pastured, allowed to graze, peck and forage all day, are best. The second best and still a good option are animals who are fed organic feed.

Additional factors in our physical environments, such as chemicals in our food and water, as well as certain other foods, can cause food sensitivities and allergies, which can cause mental and emotional symptoms, weight gain, the development of degenerative conditions and rapid ageing. Some of the worst offenders are milk products and all convenience and industrially processed packaged food. These, too, are considered low vibrational foods. This diet bears a similarity to a raw food and plant-based diets since higher vibrations are gained mostly from raw foods.

Some diets can be viewed as extreme, particularly the raw food diet, where no cooked food is consumed. However, being mindful of what you consume on a daily basis and ensuring that most of your meals are eaten in their natural state will help increase your daily intake of nutrients.

But nutrients are not all that we get from food. There is another aspect we need to consider, particularly as we go through The Change. Food affects our minds because it literally alters our bodies' chemistry.

As my interest in nutrition developed, I found that most of my conversations centred on this subject, even if this was not my intention. What I discovered from numerous interactions is that those who ate more natural foods felt more harmonious with nature, and by eating consciously, they developed an awareness of their own inner sensitivity. Furthermore, they were more observant of their food choices and how they felt after eating various foods. Developing this cognisance whilst going through The Change is necessary if we want to reduce or eliminate uncomfortable symptoms and achieve homeostasis.

The energy of natural food changes the vibration of your nervous system and is calming and healing to the soul. More information is coming to light about the vibration of food as people start to look to nature and a plant-based diet for healing. I came across a research study in the *British Journal of Cancer* that found that vegans have a 16% higher testosterone level than their carnivorous peers (Allen et al., 2000).

By eating consciously, you will begin to feel the benefits both mentally and physically. I am not advocating that you adopt a vegan diet, but I do encourage you to make sure that your plate consists mainly of natural foods and organic fresh foods and that you make an effort to purchase meat that is grass-fed or organic to reduce the amount of pesticides, additives and hormones in your meals. As they say, Rome was not built in a day, so take your time and enjoy the process. Be creative with your meals. You may have to shop around for grass-fed meat, but some local supermarkets now stock organic eggs and chicken, which indicates that food manufacturers are listening to public concerns about the effect of certain foods on health.

CHAPTER 9

NUTRITION –
THE KEY TO ACHIEVING VITALITY

When I studied raw food nutrition, I was going through a lifestyle change. I tried many different diets in the past, primarily to lose weight, but I had long given up as I ended up putting on more weight than I lost. Now that I am menopausal, shifting stubborn fat is difficult but not impossible. Like many of my friends, my first thought was hormone replacement therapy, although I knew of the possible health implications of such treatment. However, having completed this course of study, I began to look more into nutrition as a way of managing the menopause. After all, proper nutrition supplies the building blocks for life, and it is now becoming the preferred option for many when treating disease or improving homeostasis in the body.

The discovery of the chemical nature of foods, carbohydrates, fats and proteins came to the forefront of science in the 20th century. As society became increasingly aware and concerned about how nutrition affects our health, the fields of nutrition and alternative medicine saw unprecedented growth and expansion. Eating a balanced diet is vital for good health and wellbeing, and we need a wide variety of different foods to provide the right amounts of nutrients for good health, even more so as we age (University of Washington, n.d.). I have included a section on supplements as a guide to what your body requires during this transition that will start you on your way to better health.

Changing how we eat can be somewhat daunting as most of us have formed dietary habits from our childhood, culture and lifestyle, and these are habits that we might not want to change. I recall when, a few years into becoming a vegetarian, I attended a family gathering, and I sat at the dinner table, fighting the urge to tuck into the meat dishes. I could practically taste the flavours and, for a second, had food envy as I watched everyone else tuck into their meat. My plate of vegetables, rice and beans appeared to be lacking. My conscience soon nudged me back to my senses, reminding me of why I'd changed my diet, and my health was improving because of the changes I had made. My allergies were a distant memory and my menopausal symptoms were reducing. That was enough motivation to resist the urge to go back to eating the way I used to. You might face similar challenges as you make changes to your diet, but don't give up. The rewards of feeling and looking amazing are worth it. The hormonal changes we experience prior to and during this transition can be stressful to our bodies, and our nutritional needs increase with age. This is the primary reason why we have to change dietary habits to ensure our bodies are getting sufficient nutrients and to reduce the risk of age-related diseases. For normal physiology, you need to consume high quality, nutrient-dense foods like organic fruit and vegetables and grass-fed meat. Whilst studying as a natural chef I learnt about foods that are rich in phytoestrogens and are highly recommended at this stage of your life for their effectiveness in counteracting symptoms associated with the menopause.

We have now established that increasing your intake of vegetables is highly recommended as they bring the light and energy they absorb and store through photosynthesis into your body. Eating these foods in season optimises their nutritional benefits. We can also benefit immensely from including these types of foods in our diets regardless of age, but even more so as our bodies adjust during The Change. By consuming foods rich in phytoestrogen we nourish our bodies and, in turn, boost our energy levels. You can make a start now by reducing or avoiding genetically modified foods, corn, canola and cottonseed oils, processed sugar and ultra processed foods as they lack light energy. Our bodies struggle to communicate, digest and utilise these foods, a consequence of which is illnesses. It's called 'junk food' for a reason. Foods containing monosodium glutamate, yeast extract, glutamic acid, gelatin, barley malt, corn starch, soya sauce, unspecified seasonings, whey protein, added gluten and artificial flavours are neurotoxins used by the food industry to make food taste good and extend shelf-life. They overexcite the cells, affect hormones and can also cause hypertension (Cristy's Kitchen, 2024). Unfortunately, most of us consume foods that contain these additives in excess throughout most of our lives, not knowing the potential detriment to our health.

Changing your diet can seem daunting, primarily because we have attachments to food, whether psychological or physiological. Food not only nourishes us but comforts us in times of stress. Food is social as it brings people together, but we need to make wise choices as we go through The Change. When starting out making changes to your diet, start small. Begin by replacing processed foods with fresh foods. Try to eat food in its natural state and limit the amount of powdered seasoning you add to your dishes as you now know that not all seasonings are good for you due to their high sodium content, which can elevate your blood pressure. Blood pressure is known as the silent killer because symptoms are often not recognised. Managing blood pressure can become an issue for some people going through The Change. Powdered seasonings such as turmeric, fenugreek, cinnamon and oregano are beneficial for blood pressure. For example, oregano is a powerful antioxidant, as well as turmeric, which also contains anti-inflammatory properties. Cinnamon also helps lower blood sugar levels, helping your cells respond better to insulin. Try fresh herbs to add flavour to your meal, and cut back on table salt.

Here are some simple changes you can make to your diet:

- Swap ultra processed foods for healthier versions.

- Use agave nectar or honey instead of sugar.

- Eat wholegrain bread instead of white bread.

- Swap white flour for ancient grain flours such as spelt flour. Spelt flour has more soluble fibre, which is good for circulation.

- Substitute caffeinated beverages for herbal teas. Lemon balm tea, for example, is very calming and lemongrass tea is good for cleansing. If you feel fatigued, a cup of liquorice tea is a good energiser. Cinnamon tea is warming for those cold evenings. Mint tea is very cooling and aids digestion. Most supermarkets now stock these teas. (Check with your health care practitioner when buying herbal teas as some herbal supplements are contraindicated with certain medications).

- Non-GMO soya is a good alternative to meat. It's an excellent source of protein, fibre, vitamins and minerals, as well as the other health properties I mentioned earlier. Soya does not contain the saturated fat and cholesterol found in meat.

Soya is, however, one of the most contested products in supermarkets because it contains phytoestrogens that mimic the body's natural estrogen. Soya may also increase the growth of estrogen-dependent cancers such as breast cancer. However, soya beans and soya-based products such as tofu benefit cardiovascular health, weight loss and the prevention of certain other types of cancer. This can be confusing for us when deciding on whether we should include soya as a staple in our diets. Women in Asia eat soya as their main source of protein and in far greater quantities than Westerners. Meat is not eaten as much as in the West, reducing the over-consumption of unhealthy animal fat and added hormones. It is, however, possible that the latter is responsible for the increased risk to health. It is also possible that more processed soya products, such as veggie burgers and veggie hot dogs, are not as beneficial as the less processed soya products, such as tofu and tempeh, traditionally consumed in Asia, which could also be a contributing factor. Given the emerging information around soya, it is advisable that if you're at risk for hormone-sensitive conditions such as breast or ovarian cancer, speak to your health advisor or nutritionist before including soya in your diet. Healthy food is fuel for your body. Choosing to eat nutritiously will give you stamina, vitality, help with weight management and foster wellbeing. Expand your palate with more plant-based cuisine. There are so many gourmet plant-based recipes online that you can create at home, and I have included a few in this book.

There is so much talk about superfoods nowadays, and yes, they are beneficial. People who have added these foods to their diets have experienced marvelous results. However, do not overlook local foods that are just as nutritious and readily available. Berries are grown and cultivated right here in the United Kingdom. Like me, you might have ignored them as you passed them on the way to the health shop to stock up on the latest superfood, but berries are superfoods in their own right. Packed with antioxidants called anthocyanins, a type of flavonoid, berries offer anti-inflammatory, anti-viral and anticancer benefits. They also contain higher levels of a variety of phytochemicals than other fruits, which protects against DNA damage and reduces the risk of oxidative stress mediated diseases such as neurodegenerative and heart damage (Golovinskaia & Wang, 2021).

- Berries contain phytoestrogens, which are great for hormonal symptoms such as premenstrual tension, bloating and food cravings. They also provide relief for hot flashes

- A cupful of blueberries and strawberries can slow mental decline as we age, reduce blood pressure and improve cardiovascular health. This is definitely a bonus in my book. These marvellous berries also provide you with soluble and insoluble fibre (Harvard Health, 2013). Blueberries also contain tryptophan, the precursor to serotonin, so they help you sleep (UCI, 2022).

- Raspberries are equally as powerful. They have anticancer effects and are a good source of vitamin K, which helps increase bone mineral density. Raspberries may be able to reduce the risk of obesity as well as the risk of fatty liver (Burton-Freeman et al., 2016).

- We should not forget blackberries. Blackberries are one of the fruits richest in omega-3 fatty acids. A one cup serving of blackberries contains 135 milligrams of omega-3 fatty acids per serving (Cibdol, 2023).

- Goji Berries are a powerful antioxidant that boosts the immune system and is good for your eyes and skin. These berries also increase testosterone (Carey, 2023).

There is a lot of research about the benefits of cranberries for urinary tract infections, but did you know that they are also packed with proanthocyanidins, which raise the overall antioxidant capacity in our bloodstream and help reduce the risk of oxidative stress, keeping the heart healthy (Ware, 2023). Cranberries also enhance oral health which is important during menopause as less estrogen can cause gum sensitivity and gum disease which may lead to tooth loss. Incorporate berries in your daily diet as you go through The Change. The benefits are unquestionable and will immensely reduce your risk of degenerative diseases as you go through this transition. You can add berries to your smoothies or cereal or freeze them and eat them as a snack. Not only will they add flavour, but they will also make your meals more interesting and tastier.

As well as eating food to manage your symptoms, you might want to consider using herbs. Herbs can be an effective and safe alternative to pharmaceutical drugs, and they have a lot of medicinal properties. Many people are turning to herbs because they are concerned about the side effects of chemically altering their physiology through medicine. This was one of the reasons I did not pursue hormone replacement therapy and turned to nature instead.

CHAPTER 10

Therapeutic Meals for a Smoother Transition

To say menopause presents us with many challenges is an understatement. You start to look and feel differently due to having lower hormone levels and what you eat on a daily basis likely has an impact on your symptoms. Therefore, it is important for you to eat food that will help balance your hormones. Furthermore, your body requires more or less of certain foods. For example, as you no longer have a monthly cycle, you won't need as much iron in your diet. The risk of osteoporosis increases in menopause, and many women end up with fractures when they fall. Given these changes, menopause really is a good time to review your diet. Even more so, as you might have picked up poor eating habits over the years and probably have a lot of toxins in your body, which can cause more intense menopause symptoms. What you put on your plate can either intensify or reduce symptoms. In chapter 9, I went into detail on how certain food can trigger or intensify certain symptoms. You might recall that for some women, consuming alcohol or eating spicy food can trigger hot flashes, and some women find that eating chocolate triggers headaches since they've started the menopause. For me, the weight gain was the bane of my menopause journey. I only had to look at a packet of crisps or candy, and I could feel the weight piling on. I gained a lot of fat around the abdomen due to my hormones and unhealthy eating habits, and I had to learn to stop eating for pleasure and comfort, change my relationship with food, and eat more mindfully. In the meal plan on the following page, I include a lot of raw and plant-based foods that have not been pasteurised or homogenised because our bodies find them easier to digest as they are not as hard to process as meat, fish, dairy and grains, although these foods are also nutritious. Additional benefits of consuming mainly plant-based meals include improved metabolism and digestion, better weight control and more energy as you flood your body with life-sustaining oxygen and antioxidants from plants. Plants are rich in phytoestrogens, helping balance hormones. I have included some tasty recipes in the meal plan to help you reduce some of the more uncomfortable symptoms.

Let's look at a few examples of how you can use food to eradicate or reduce symptoms. If you experience low libido, poor memory and concentration or a loss of motivation, increasing your intake of avocados, chia seeds and bananas will boost your testosterone levels. Herbs such as Fadogia agrestis are especially beneficial in boosting testosterone levels and also help men who experience erectile dysfunction while going through andropause. Getting in your 'five a day' can be a struggle at times, and this is where juicing comes in handy. You can pack a lot of fruit and vegetables into your juicer to get your daily amount. I have included a few juice recipes in the meal plan. Juicing is also beneficial for detoxifying the liver, which may contain excess hormones. If you experience weight gain, dry skin or rashes, irritability, or insomnia your liver might be congested. Vegetable broth is a great way to get in your daily count of vegetables. Using vegetables rich in potassium will help regulate blood pressure, which can increase during menopause. Mushrooms are also good for keeping your blood pressure down because they're low in sodium. They are also a great source of selenium, which helps thyroid function. Shitake mushrooms contain copper, which helps with declining collagen production as you age. Collagen helps with elasticity and hydration, preventing the skin on your face from sagging. It also improves bone, ligaments and joints, as well as slowing the greying of hair. If you are not keen on mushrooms, consider using copper utensils to help your body produce more collagen. These therapeutic meals are protein-rich to help maintain lean muscle, which is important as we lose muscle mass as we age. It's also anti-inflammatory and high in antioxidants to start you on the road to a healthier menopause transition.

You don't have to follow this meal plan as it's presented; you can mix it up and change some of the ingredients if you choose. Some of these meals are my creations, while others have been adapted from my training as a raw food nutritionist and natural chef. I found that my health improved immensely since changing my diet. Changing your diet does not have to be costly or difficult. Getting back to basics is the key to being healthy and reducing symptoms during menopause. These meals are not complicated, and if you are busy as I am most of the time you can make batches of soups, juices and smoothies ahead of time and pop them in the freezer, which will help preserve the nutrients. I hope you enjoy them.

Meal Plan

	Breakfast	Lunch	Dinner
Sunday	Chia Seeds pancakes	Meal of your choice	Roast Turkey and Root vegetables
Monday	Watermelon Salad	Chickpea Crepes with creamy Mushrooms & Spinach	Pine Nut Pesto Pasta
Tuesday	Green Goddess Juice	Potassium Broth	Mexican Vegan Stew with Quinoa
Wednesday	Super Green Smoothie	Chicken and Avocado Sandwich	Mushroom Risotto
Thursday	Vegan Egg -free Benedict	Butternut Squash with sweet Potato soup	Garden Salad
Friday	Raw Cacoa Maca Moca Smoothie	Veggie with Hummus sandwich	Vegetable Kebab
Saturday	Scrambled Tofu, Tomatoes	Kale Salad, roasted sweet potato	Poached salmon, Quinoa and Spinach

Recipes

Chia Seed Pancakes

Ingredients

- *375 g organic oat flour (you can make your own by blending rolled oats)*
- *1 large overripe banana, mashed*
- *1 tsp baking powder*
- *1 tsp flaxseeds*
- *2 tbsp pure maple syrup*
- *1 tsp vanilla extract*
- *1 chia seed 'egg' (add 1 tbsp chia seeds and 3 tbsp water to a separate bowl. Let sit to thicken)*
- *250 g dairy-free milk of choice*

Instructions

1. Mix flaxseeds, oat flour and baking powder in large mixing bowl.
2. Mash banana and add to mixing bowl.
3. Add maple syrup, vanilla and chia egg to flour mixture.
4. Add milk and let sit to thicken if batter seems runny.
5. Heat large, non-stick frying pan to high temperature (if your frying pan tends to stick, use a little bit of coconut oil or vegan butter to coat pan).
6. Add about 1/3 cup of batter to hot pan for each pancake. When edges show a few bubbles, they are ready to flip.

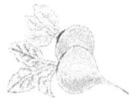

Watermelon Fruit Salad

Ingredients

- *1000 g watermelon, chopped into bite-sized chunks*
- *200 g sweet cherries, pitted and halved*
- *200 g blueberries*
- *1½ tbsp fresh lime juice*
- *1 tbsp light agave nectar*
- *1/4 tsp lime zest*
- *2 tsp fresh mint*

Instructions

1. Place fresh fruit in large bowl.
2. In small bowl, mix lime juice and agave and pour over salad.

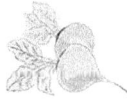

Green Goddess Juice

Ingredients

- *1 kale leaf*
- *1 green apple (preferably with skin)*
- *1/4 inch ginger root*
- *4 large celery sticks*
- *1 cucumber, roughly chopped*
- *1/2 lemon*
- *Handful fresh parsley*
- *1 tsp wheatgrass*

Instructions

1. Juice all ingredients except wheatgrass in order presented.
2. Pour into glass.
3. Add 1 tsp wheatgrass and stir in glass until dissolved.

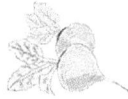

Raw Cacao Maca Mocha Smoothie

Ingredients

- 65 g raspberries
- 3 Brazil nuts
- 1 tbsp hemp seeds or linseeds
- 2 tbsp raw cacao/carob powder
- 1 tsp maca powder.
- 1 tsp raw honey
- 200 ml almond or coconut milk
- Ice cubes

Instructions

1. Add raspberries to blender with all ingredients except ice.
2. Blend until smooth.
3. Towards end of process, add small amount of ice and blend again if you want an ice-cold drink.

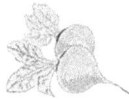

Scrambled Tofu and Tomato (serves 2)

Ingredients

- 1 tomato
- 1 tbsp olive oil
- 1 tsp red wine vinegar
- 1/4 tsp Himalayan salt (or other natural salt)
- 1/4 tbsp black pepper, freshly ground
- 1 tsp garlic powder
- 1 tsp dried mixed herbs (like an Italian blend)
- 1 tsp ground turmeric
- 300 g extra-firm tofu, drained
- 1/2 yellow onion, finely diced
- 1 zucchini, diced
- 1/2 red bell pepper, diced
- 2 tbsp nutritional yeast

Instructions

1. Preheat oven to 400° F/ 204° C.
2. Quarter tomato and cut each quarter in half, crosswise.
3. In medium bowl, toss tomato, 1 tsp olive oil, vinegar, salt and pepper.
4. Transfer to baking sheet and bake until soft and slightly caramelised, 25–30 minutes.
5. In medium mixing bowl, combine garlic powder, dried herbs and turmeric. Crumble tofu in bowl and mix to combine. Set aside
6. Heat large skillet/frying pan over medium heat. Add onion and remaining 1 tsp oil and sauté onion until soft and translucent.
7. Add zucchini and bell pepper; cook until tender.
8. Add tofu and nutritional yeast and cook, stirring often until heated through, about 4 minutes.
9. Serve with roasted tomatoes.

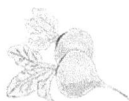

Vegan Eggs Benedict (serves 2)

Ingredients

- *Whole grain muffins*
- *300 g medium or soft tofu, cut into thick slices*
- *1 avocado*
- *Juice of 1 large lemon*
- *1 tsp Dijon mustard*
- *1 tsp Cajun seasoning*
- *1 tbsp coconut oil plus more for grilling and baking*
- *Salt and pepper to taste*
- *4 spears of asparagus*
- *1 tsp apple cider vinegar*
- *Vegan hollandaise (recipe to follow)*

Instructions

1. Press tofu with tofu press or place on plate, wrap in paper towel and press firmly until water drains from tofu. You can place a pile of books on the tofu instead, and leave for 10 minutes.
2. Once drained, pat each side of each piece with paper towel, then brush each side with olive oil and season with a pinch of salt, pepper and Cajun seasoning.
3. Leave to marinate for 2 hours or overnight.
4. Preheat grill and oven.
5. Place asparagus in a large bowl. Pour oil and vinegar over them and toss to coat evenly.
6. Spread asparagus spears in single layer on baking tray. Bake for 20 minutes in preheated oven or until tender and bright green.
7. Whilst asparagus is roasting, grill tofu pieces for approximately 10 minutes (5 minutes on each side) until they begin to brown.
8. Cut muffins in half and toast until tops are golden brown and crispy.
9. Top muffins with Hollandaise sauce and build up a staff with asparagus and tofu.

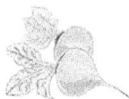

Avocado Hollandaise Sauce

Ingredients

- *1 avocado, peeled and pitted*
- *Juice of 1 lemon*
- *Water to get the right consistency*
- *Salt and pepper to taste*

Instructions

Puree avocado, lemon juice and salt in blender until smooth, adding just enough water to make sauce creamy and thick like a real hollandaise.

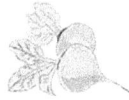

Kale Salad (serves 2)

Ingredients

- 1 head kale, torn into small pieces
- 1 thick slice fresh pineapple, cubed
- 1 avocado, cubed
- 1/2 red onion, thinly sliced
- 3 dates, pitted and roughly torn

Dressing ingredients

- 2 tbsp olive oil
- 2 tbsp toasted sesame oil
- 3 tbsp apple cider vinegar
- 1/2 tsp Celtic sea salt, coarsely ground
- Pinch of black pepper

Instructions

Toss all dressing ingredients first, then toss salad ingredients in a large bowl and pour dressing over salad. Toss again.

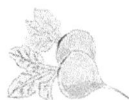

Savoury Roasted Sweet Potato

Ingredients

- *1 large sweet potato, peeled and diced*
- *1 tbsp rapeseed oil*
- *Cumin, coriander and cayenne pepper to taste*

Instructions

1. Preheat oven to 400° F/205° C.
2. Place potato in bowl and drizzle with oil. Sprinkle cumin, coriander and cayenne pepper over potato.
3. Mix with hands until potato is well coated.
4. Placed diced sweet potato evenly on a baking sheet in one layer.
5. Bake for 30 minutes or until potato is tender.

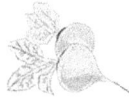

Potassium Broth (serves 2)

Ingredients

- *750 ml water*
- *125 g carrots*
- *125 g broccoli*
- *125 g butternut squash*
- *62 g mushrooms*
- *2 celery stalks*
- *2 tbsp diced parsley*
- *8 fresh tomatoes*
- *1 onion, diced*
- *2 garlic cloves, finely chopped*
- *1/4 tsp dried basil*

Instructions

1. Liquefy tomatoes in blender.
2. Combine ingredients in soup pot and bring to boil for 30 minutes.
3. Strain and serve.

Note

You can reserve vegetables for another recipe. Mash and eat with a little butter or put in a smoothie.

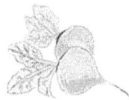

Chicken and Avocado Sandwich

Ingredients

2 slices wholegrain bread, lightly toasted

- *1 small chicken breast, poached and shredded*
- *2 medium egg yolks*
- *1 avocado large and very ripe, mashed until smooth*
- *1 tsp mustard*
- *Sea salt to taste*
- *Lemon juice, freshly squeezed*
- *1/2 red onion, sliced*
- *1 handful rocket*

Instructions

1. Make mayonnaise with pestle and mortar by mashing avocado into egg yolks.
2. Season with sea salt, mustard and lemon juice to taste.
3. Fold in chicken.
4. Layer rocket on toasted bread, then chicken, avocado and mayonnaise followed by pinch of black pepper before layering onion slices.

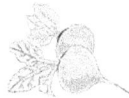

Veggie and Hummus Sandwich

Ingredients

- *4 slices wholegrain bread*
- *Hummus*
- *Fresh spinach leaves*
- *1 large carrot, grated*
- *1 large ripe tomato, sliced*
- *1 ripe avocado, sliced*
- *1 red onion, thinly sliced*
- *Alfalfa sprouts*
- *Salt and pepper to taste*

Instructions

1. Add thick layer of hummus to inside of each slice of bread.
2. On two slices of bread, add thin layer of fresh spinach leaves.
3. Top with grated carrot, then tomato slices.
4. Add salt and pepper to tomato slices, then add avocado and red onion and a sprinkle of alfalfa sprouts
5. Add second slice of bread, hummus side down. Slice in half and serve right away.

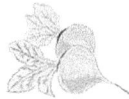

Chickpea Crepes with Creamy Mushrooms & Spinach (serves 2)

Ingredients

- *160 g chickpea flour*
- *240 ml water*
- *Pinch each of salt and pepper*
- *1 small onion, finely chopped or grated*
- *3 garlic cloves, minced*
- *1 tbsp mixed herbs*
- *Rapeseed oil*

Filling ingredients

- *Rapeseed oil*
- *300 g mushrooms, sliced*
- *2 handfuls spinach*
- *Vegan cream cheese*
- *Water*

Instructions for Chickpea Flour

Place dried chickpeas in high-speed blender. Pulse several times until chickpeas are broken down into fine powder and a flour begins to form. You will need to make (or purchase) 160 g chickpea flour.

Crepes

1. In medium bowl, mix together chickpea flour and water. Don't worry if the mixture is a bit lumpy or thin.
2. Stir in remaining ingredients and leave to sit for 19 minutes.
3. Meanwhile, heat up your crepe maker (heat setting 4) or non-stick frying pan, brushed with small amount of oil.
4. Add a ¼ cup of mixture and pour into pan or crepe maker, adding more mixture if needed to cover the base of the crepe maker or frying pan.

5. Cook for approximately 4 minutes before gently flipping and cooking the other side until golden brown.
6. Repeat with the rest of the mixture

Instructions for Filling

1. Drizzle rapeseed oil in pan and cook sliced mushrooms on medium heat for a few minutes until lightly browned and softened.
2. Add spinach, stir well, and allow to cook down.
3. Add a few dollops of vegan cheese and stir everything together. Add a drop of water if too thick.
4. Allow to simmer for a couple of minutes to heat through.
5. Add dollop of filling to each crepe and roll and spread across the surface. Roll crepes, plate and serve.

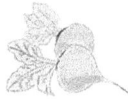

Butternut Squash & Sweet Potato Soup (serves 2)

Ingredients
- *1 tsp coconut oil*
- *1 red onion, roughly chopped*
- *2 carrots, roughly chopped*
- *1 sweet potato, diced*
- *1 medium size butternut squash, diced*
- *1 zucchini diced*
- *1 clove of garlic, crushed*
- *1 leak, roughly chopped*
- *1 litre vegetable stock*
- *1 tsp whole black peppercorn (optional)*
- *Sea salt to taste*

Instructions
1. Heat coconut oil in large pan over medium heat and gently sauté onions for 5 minutes.
2. Add garlic, stir and cook for a further 2 minutes.
3. Add carrot, sweet potato, leak and zucchini and stir intermittently until slightly caramelised.
4. Add vegetable stock and stir soup, mixing everything together.
5. Simmer on low heat for 20 minutes (depending on how soft you like your vegetables).
6. Once vegetables have softened, remove from stove and let cool for 10 minutes. Ladle soup into blender or food processor and pulse to a smooth puree or leave slightly chunky, if you prefer.

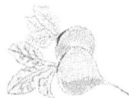

Grilled Salmon with Quinoa and Sautéed Spinach
(serves 2)

Ingredients
- *2 fillets salmon*
- *1/4 tsp pepper*
- *1/4 tsp garlic powder*
- *Pinch of salt*
- *43 g brown sugar*
- *3 tbsp of water*
- *3 tbsp of soy sauce*
- *2 tbsp of rapeseed oil*
- *3 cloves of garlic*
- *2 shallots*

Ingredients for Quinoa
- *250 ml vegetable broth or water*
- *1/2 tsp sea salt*
- *1 tbsp unsalted butter*
- *250 g quinoa*

Ingredients for Spinach
- *Generous handful spinach*
- *1 tbsp rapeseed oil*

Instructions for Grilling Salmon
1. Season salmon fillets with pepper, garlic powder and salt.
2. In small bowl, stir together soy sauce, brown sugar, water and rapeseed oil until sugar has dissolved.
3. Pour sauce over salmon. Cover and refrigerate for at least 2 hours.
4. Preheat grill on medium heat. Lightly oil grill grate.
5. Place salmon on preheated grill and discard marinade. Cook salmon for 6–8 minutes per side or until the fish flakes easily with a fork.
6. Set aside to cool.

Instructions for Quinoa

1. In medium saucepan, bring water or broth, salt and butter to boil.
2. Stir in quinoa. Cover with lid and reduce heat to simmer for 10–15 minutes.

Instructions for Spinach

1. Heat 2 tbsp rapeseed oil in large skillet on medium high heat. Add spinach to pan.
2. Cover pan and cook for 1 minute.
3. Uncover and turn spinach over.
4. Cover pan and cook for an additional minute.
5. Remove from heat.

Assemble plate

Place quinoa on plate and flatten to spread out. Layer spinach and 1 salmon fillet on each plate. Serve.

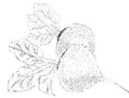

Garden Salad (serves 2)

Ingredients

- *160 g mixed lettuce*
- *25 g zucchini, julienned*
- *1 Medjool date, torn roughly into pieces*
- *2 pieces dried mango, roughly chopped*
- *1/2 small avocado, peeled and sliced*
- *1/4 red onion, thinly sliced*
- *4 fresh basil leaves, finely chopped*

Dressing ingredients

- *2 tbsp lemon juice*
- *1 tsp olive oil*
- *Pinch of fresh ground pepper*

Instructions

1. Fill plate with green lettuce.
2. Toss remaining ingredients and top lettuce.
3. Mix dressing ingredients in jar and shake well.
4. Pour dressing over salad and serve immediately.

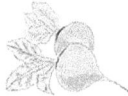

Mexican Stew (serves 2)

Ingredients

- 1 tbsp rapeseed oil
- 1/2 red onion
- 1 red chilli pepper, deseeded and finely sliced
- 1 plump garlic clove, finely chopped
- 1 yellow pepper, deseeded and chopped
- 1 tsp paprika
- 1 tsp tomato puree
- 200 ml vegetable stock
- 1 x 400 g tin black beans, drained
- 1 x 400 g pinto beans, drained
- 50 g butternut squash, diced
- 180 g quinoa
- 250 ml water
- 3 spring onions, thinly sliced
- 1 tsp chilli powder
- 1 tsp ground turmeric
- 2 tbsp nutritional yeast
- 20 g fresh coriander, finely chopped

Instructions

1. Heat oil in pan over medium heat and sauté onion and chillies for 3 minutes.
2. Add garlic and yellow peppers and cook for 5 minutes.
3. Stir in paprika, nutritional yeast and tomato puree.
4. Add vegetable stock, drained beans and squash.
5. After 5 minutes, reduce heat to simmer.

Instructions for quinoa

1. Bring water or broth, salt and butter to boil in medium saucepan.
2. Stir in quinoa. Cover with lid and reduce heat to simmer for 10–15 minutes.

3. Remove from heat. Use fork to fluff and separate grains.
4. Fold in spring onions, chilli powder and ground turmeric.
5. Spoon quinoa into large serving dish or platter. Spoon vegetable and bean mix over or alongside mixture.
6. Scatter coriander over top. Serve.

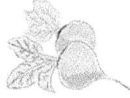

Vegan Kebabs

- *5 cherry tomatoes*
- *1/2 zucchini*
- *1/2 red bell pepper*
- *1/2 yellow pepper*
- *1 red onion*
- *240 g extra firm tofu*
- *1 thick slice pineapple*
- *2 tbsp toasted sesame oil*
- *Sea salt*
- *Black pepper*
- *4 wooden skewers*

Ingredients for dipping sauce

- *2 tbsp tamari sauce*
- *2 tbsp maple syrup*
- *1/4 tsp chilli powder*
- *1/4 tsp garlic powder*
- *2 tbsp hot water*

Instructions

1. Place skewers in shallow dish, cover with water and allow to soak for 15 minutes.
2. Cut tofu into large pieces. Place on parchment-lined baking tray and place in oven to bake at 460° F (240° C) for 15 minutes.
3. Chop bell peppers and zucchini into thick, large slices.
4. Chop pineapple slice into large chunks.
5. Toss chopped veg and cherry tomatoes in bowl. Add 2 tbsp sesame oil, sea salt and black pepper. Toss together so everything is coated.
6. Remove tofu from oven and brush with remaining 1 tbsp sesame oil.

7. Thread vegetables and tofu onto skewers and place on a parchment-lined baking tray.
8. Place into the oven and bake at 350° F (180° C) for 30 minutes.

Instructions for dipping sauce

Add hot water, soy sauce, maple syrup, chili and garlic spices together and whisk to combine. Serve vegetable skewers with bowl of dipping sauce on the side

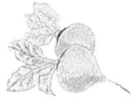

Pine Nut Pesto Pasta

Ingredients

- *250 g wholegrain fettuccine or spaghetti*
- *1 tsp light cream to taste*
- *125 g frozen peas*
- *125 g packet raw pine nuts*
- *1 large clove garlic, finely chopped*
- *2 tbsp rapeseed oil*
- *25 g mint or basil leaves, firmly packed*
- *1 tsp sea salt*
- *1 tsp black pepper, freshly ground*

Instructions

1. Place frozen peas in bowl.
2. Cook pasta in plenty of boiling water until al dente.
3. When cooked, do not discard water. Pour over frozen peas to thaw.
4. Drain peas. Place in food processor with pine nuts and garlic and coarsely blend.
5. Scrape down sides. Add oil, choice of herbs and salt.
6. Blend again to a medium-thick paste.
7. Season well with pepper.
8. Spoon into saucepan with pasta. Using 2 spoons, toss over medium heat, slowly adding cream until heated through.

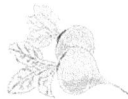

Mushroom Risotto (serves 4)

Ingredients

- *250 g brown rice*
- *Spray oil*
- *1 red onion, finely chopped*
- *3 cloves garlic, sliced*
- *280 g mushrooms*
- *2 tsp brown miso*
- *1 tsp ground cumin*
- *250 g silken tofu*
- *32 g flaxseed*

Instructions

1. Bring 0.5 litres water to boil and add rice.
2. Reduce heat to simmer, cover and cook for 50 minutes.
3. Spray (or wipe) heavy frying pan with oil. Heat over medium-high heat.
4. Sauté onion, garlic and mushroom until browned.
5. Reduce heat to low, add cooked rice and stir.
6. Puree miso, cumin and tofu in food processor with the S-blade inserted.
7. Add rice and mushroom mix. Stir.
8. Add flaxseed. Cook uncovered for 5 minutes without boiling.

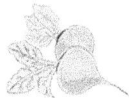

Roasted Turkey and Vegetables (serves 4)

Instructions

- *Whole turkey, giblets removed*
- *Few sprigs each of fresh thyme, oregano, sage and parsley*
- *1 tbsp rapeseed oil*
- *1 tsp dry white wine*
- *1 tsp paprika*
- *Fresh ground pepper*
- *1 small orange, peeled and cut into wedges*
- *1 onion, cut into wedges*
- *125 ml chicken broth*

Ingredients for Roasted Vegetables

- *1 fennel bulb*
- *2 large carrots*
- *1 parsnip*
- *1 raw beetroot*
- *2 tbsp rapeseed oil*
- *Few sprigs of rosemary*
- *Sprinkle of sea salt flakes*

Instructions for Turkey

1. Lift up skin covering turkey breast. Slip thyme, oregano, sage and parsley underneath skin, spread out evenly.
2. Combine oil, wine, paprika and pepper. Rub mixture over surface of turkey.
3. Place oranges and onions inside turkey.
4. Place turkey in roasting pan, breast side down.
5. Pour chicken broth into bottom of pan.
6. Cover loosely with aluminium foil.
7. Preheat oven to 325° F/162° C/Gas 3.
8. Roast 20–25 minutes per pound, basting periodically.
9. Halfway through cooking, flip turkey, breast-side up.

10. During last 25 minutes of roasting, remove foil cover.
11. Continue to roast until leg moves easily and juices run clear.
12. Let stand for 20 minutes to let juices settle for easier carving.

Instructions for Roasting Vegetables

1. Heat oven to 220° C/420° F/Gas 7.
2. Cut vegetables into evenly sized wedges.
3. Toss all vegetables with olive oil and put into large roasting tin. Top with thyme springs.
4. Bake in oven until tender, about 40–50 minutes.
5. Sprinkle with sea salt and serve at once.

Note

You will have to time the roasting of your vegetables with the turkey. Put vegetables in oven approximately 1 hour before turkey is ready to be removed from oven.

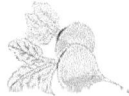

CHAPTER 11

HERBS AND SUPPLEMENTS

And God said, "Behold, I have given you every herb bearing seed,
which is upon the face of all the earth, and every tree, in the which
{is} the fruit of a tree yielding seed; to you it shall be for meat"
(Genesis 1:29 King James Version)

Plants have been used for medicinal purposes since time began. Hippocrates (the 'father of medicine'), Herophilos and Erasistratus studied herbal medicine at the temple of Amenhotep in ancient Egypt and brought herbal medicine to Greece, which later spread across Asia and Europe. In some Asian and African countries, a large percentage of the population still rely on herbs as medicine for their primary health care needs. Many modern prescription medications are inspired by or derived from natural plant chemicals. As people search for healthier lifestyles, they are rediscovering the medicinal properties of herbs. The rise in herbalism, natural products, complimentary therapies, raw food and plant-based cuisine attests to the demand for more natural lifestyles as people take more responsibility for their health and wellbeing. The United Kingdom's expenditure on complementary or alternative medicine increase yearly as more people turn to herbal medicine to complement or replace conventional medicine. I chose the path of herbal medicine in 2008 when I was having a terrible time with uterine fibroids. They caused me so much distress: heavy menstruation, abdominal cramps and even urine retention. I recall having to go to the Accident and Emergency Department at my local hospital on at least two occasions in the middle of the night because I couldn't pee; a fibroid had grown so large that it was pressing on my bladder. It was quite mortifying. I also had to leave my place of work or engagement early on many occasions because my period was so heavy.

A friend of mine introduced me to a naturopathic consultant who prescribed herbs, a liver cleanse, a course of colonics and a detox, which consisted of a juice fast and eliminating meat products. Within a few months, a scan revealed that my fibroids stopped growing and my symptoms eventually lessened. I even shed a few pounds, which was a bonus. This experience sparked my interest in the use of herbs for health, particularly hormonal imbalance because that was the root cause of my health problems.

I studied herbs and their many benefits and learnt that, historically, herbs such as angelica, liquorice, chaste tree (vitex), black cohosh, ginkgo biloba and wild Mexican yam have been used for treating symptoms associated with these transformative periods in a woman's life (Echeverria et al., 2021), menopause and perimenopause and help alleviate premenstrual symptoms.

If you are considering using herbs to assist you through this transition and are taking medication, it is important to speak to your doctor or health advisor regarding possible herb-drug interactions. I have included a table of herbs in this chapter that can help manage symptoms.

As well as considering the use of herbs, you might also want to explore the use of supplements. Ever since scientists began to identify nutrients in food in the 20th century, supplements have gained widespread popularity. They can be found in most households today as a dietary addition to contribute to optimal health. Adding supplements to your diet can be beneficial for hormonal imbalances because, unless you are eating a completely raw and organic diet, most of your food is likely to lack sufficient nutrients due to improper farming practices. Even if you eat organic and raw foods, it's sometimes difficult to balance nutrition.

We are also exposed to environmental toxins and pollutants through air, water and soil, putting even more stress on our livers, kidneys, skin and lymphatic systems as they work harder to eliminate these from our bodies. The consequence is a build-up of toxins or free radicals, which damage organs, depress immune function and put us at risk of serious illnesses. Never more so than now do we need antioxidants to renovate the damage to our cells caused by free radicals. Furthermore, declining estrogen levels influence everything from bone to heart health to where and how much fat is retained and distributed throughout your body.

Below are tables that list herbs and supplements considered beneficial for hormonal imbalance as well as offering other amazing benefits. These are not conclusive as there are a wide variety of herbs and supplements available for you to choose from, but these are the ones I come across frequently, and some I still use occasionally to this day.

Fig. 1   Table of herbs

Herbs	Benefits
Agnus castus	Manages hormones. May increase progesterone levels.
Ashwagandha	Improves sleep, mood and alleviates mental exhaustion.
Black cohosh	Relieves menstrual cramps and symptoms of menopause.
Dang quai	Manages hormones and reduces fibroids, detoxifies the body, eases menstrual cramps, boosts energy levels and circulation. May increase the production of testosterone.
Ginger root	Increases circulation and promotes blood flow to the uterus.
Juniper berries	Eliminates excess water and used as a mild diuretic to treat urinary problems, usually in combination with other herbs.

Herbs	Benefits
Liquorice	Liquorice regulates hormones and could help with vaginal atrophy.
Maca root	Used for hormone management, increases libido and energy.
Marshmallow root	Lowers or prevents heartburn, stomach ulcer symptoms, diarrhoea and constipation.
Milk thistle seed	Promotes liver health.
Organic yellow dock root	A blood purifier and detoxifier, especially for the liver.
Palmetto	May be effective in reducing symptoms associated with benign prostatic hyperplasia or benign prostate enlargement.
Passionflower	May be effective in reducing anxiety.
Red clover	Red clover Reduces night sweats and has the added benefit of improving circulation.
Raspberry leaf	An antioxidant and beneficial for skin health. Also good source of iron.
Sage	Regulates the body's thermostat to reduce hot flashes. Known to improve memory.
St John's wort	Treats mild depression, mood swings and insomnia.
Valerian root	A muscle relaxant. Helps improve sleep.

Fig. 2 Table of Supplements

Supplement	Benefits
Vitamin A	A natural antioxidant that neutralises damaging free radicals. It also assists the body with the metabolism of fat
Vitamin B	Converts food to energy, supports adrenal glands and aids in the production of serotonin.
Vitamin C	As a potent antioxidant, vitamin C promotes the formation of collagen and protects against oxidative stress.
Vitamin D	Regulates insulin secretion and balances blood sugar. It may also boost testosterone levels and increase libido.
Vitamin E	An antioxidant that protects against damage to cell membranes.
Calcium	Vital for bone health and maintaining health of your teeth
Copper	Beneficial for reducing inflammation. Helpful for the protection of the skeletal, nervous and cardiovascular systems. As well as the formation of collagen
Coenzyme Q(10)	The key to your body's energy transport system, it's great for cardiovascular health and can help with hot flashes, mood swings and depression.
Glutamine	Helps repair and build muscle, helps fuel the cells that line the intestines, is an important component of the body's immune response.

Supplement	Benefits
Magnesium	Maintains normal muscle and nerve function, supports a healthy immune system and keeps bones strong. Promotes normal blood pressure and is known to be involved in many other functions.
Omega 3	Has many benefits for the health of the heart, skin and joints. It may have protective benefits against cancer.
Omega 6	Promotes healthy hair growth, rejuvenate your skin, regulates metabolism and improves bone density.
Selenium	Works with Vitamin E to prevent free radical damage to cell membranes. Selenium also increases blood flow.
Zinc	Regulates hormones and boost immune system. May also lower inflammation and stabilise mood.

I have covered a lot of information about the way in which we should eat and the herbs and supplements that may help during this phase in your life. Therefore, let me reiterate the importance of initially making small changes to your diet if you feel somewhat overwhelmed. The guidance of a health professional such as a nutritionist, natural chef, herbalist or TCM practitioner will help you to put together a tailor-made programme to make this transition easier.

Conclusion

Going through The Change need not be a stressful phase for either men or women. We have established that, through nutrition, we can manage symptoms more effectively if we take the time to examine what and how we eat. Despite advancements in the food industry, we now know that some of their practices, such as intensive farming and giving excessive growth hormones to animals, can affect us adversely and increase or intensify our symptoms. With this in mind, we need to eat more organic foods and reduce the amount of processed and non-organic foods in our diet. By doing so, we are likely to reduce illnesses linked to hormonal imbalances. This phase in life affects us not only physically but emotionally and spiritually; therefore, we should examine our attitudes towards the menopause as we undergo this phase. Your body will work at its optimum level if you take a holistic approach towards your health.

At this juncture, we embark upon one of the most crucial periods of our lives, and we need to invest time in ourselves. Use this transition to engage in meaningful activities. The menopause may signal the end of youth, but it is not the end of life. With good nutrition, mindfulness and exercise, you should still have the energy to participate in an array of activities. Having already raised your family, consider this is your time. Don't allow your hormones to dictate your quality of life.

You can follow me on Instagram or contact me by email to find out more about how you can live a healthier and more meaningful lifestyle during The Change.

About the Author

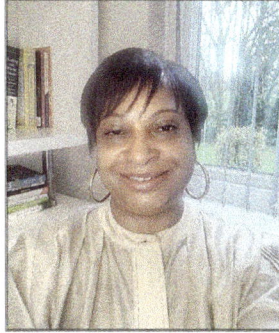

Lynette is a wellness practitioner specialising in menopause support. Her interest in nutrition and women's health began with her own experience of managing perimenopausal symptoms, which led her to study at the College of Naturopathic Medicine in London, qualifying as a Natural Chef with a focus on therapeutic menu planning.

She now works with clients to manage menopausal symptoms through targeted nutrition and lifestyle changes. Her success in helping others inspired her to write this book, offering practical, natural solutions for women and men navigating hormonal changes.

Lynette also has a long-standing background in youth justice, where she supports parents in promoting hormonal balance and emotional wellbeing in teenagers through healthy eating. She mentors young people to help them make positive life choices and acts as a mediator in families experiencing relationship breakdowns.

Contact Lynette at:
lynetteroseltd@gmail.com

Follow Lynette on Instagram:
@lynetterose_uk

References

1. Acharya, D., & Anshu, S. (2008). *Indigenous Herbal Medicines: Tribal Formulations and Traditional Herbal Practices.* Aavishkar Publishers.

2. Allen, N., Appleby, P. N., Davey, G. K., & Key, T. J. (2000, July). Hormones and diet: Low insulin-like growth factor — I but normal bioavailable androgens in vegan men. *British Journal of Cancer,* 83(1), 95–97. https://doi.org/10.1054/bjoc.2000.1152

3. Alothman, M., Hogan, S. A., Hennessy, D., Dillon, P., Kilcawley, K. N., O'Donovan, M., Tobin, J., Fenclon, M. A., & O'Callaghan, T. F. (2019, August 17). The "grass-fed" milk story: Understanding the impact of pasture feeding on the composition and quality of bovine milk. *Foods,* 8(8), 350. https://doi.org/10.3390/foods8080350

4. American Academy for Oral & Systemic Health. (2019, January 4). *Sugar, soda pop, and its impact on chronic disease.* https://www.aaosh.org/connect/sugar-soda-and-impact-on-chronic-disease

5. Animal Welfare Institute. (n.d.). *Inhumane practices on factory farms.* https://awionline.org/content/inhumane-practices-factory-farms

6. Astellas. (2024, October 18). *Silence, stigma, and misunderstanding: Our mission to break down barriers in menopause.* https://www.astellas.com/en/stories/world-menopause-day-2024

7. Atkinson, L. (2015, March 13). How to sail through the menopause: We've talked to experts and plumbed the latest research to produce the ULTIMATE guide to surviving the change. *Daily Mail*. http://www.dailymail.co.uk/health/article-2994224/ How-sail-menopause-ve-talked- experts-plumbed-latest- research-produce-ULTIMATE-book-surviving-change.html

8. Bellamy, C. (2023, October 18). *What Black women should know about hair relaxers and their health*. NBC News. https://www.nbcnews.com/news/nbcblk/black-women-hair-relaxers-cancer-rcna117685

9. Bentzen, J. S. (2021, December.) In crisis, we pray: Religiosity and the COVID-19 pandemic. Journal of *Economic Behavior & Organization*, 192, 541–583. https://doi.org/10.1016/j.jebo.2021.10.014

10. Berg. (2025, February 18). Castor oil for your face. Natures Botox. https://www.drberg.com/blog/castor-oil-for-your-face-natures-botox

11. Better Health Channel. (2022, September 12). *Fruit and vegetables*. https://www.betterhealth.vic.gov.au/health/healthyliving/fruit-and-vegetables

12. Bień, A., Niewiadomska, I., Korżyńska-Piętas. M., Rzońca, E., Zarajczyk, M., Pięta, B., & Jurek, K. (2024, August 24). General self-efficacy as a moderator between severity of menopausal symptoms and satisfaction with life in menopausal women. *Frontiers in Public Health*. https://doi.org/10.3389/fpubh.2024.1426191

13. Bockmann, M. (2021, March 18). *How to be an emotionally strong woman in relationships.* Thrive Global. https://community.thriveglobal.com/how-to-be-an-emotionally-strong-woman-in-relationships/

14. Bolland, M. J., Avenell, A., Baron, J. A., Grey, A., MacLennan, G. S., Gamble, G. D., & Reid, I. R. (2010, July 29). Effect of calcium supplements on risk of myocardial infarction and cardiovascular events: meta- analysis. *BMJ*, 341, c3691. https://doi.org/10.1136/bmj.c3691

15. Bratley, M. (2024, March 12). *Study reveals nearly one in two are worried about running out of money in retirement.* IFA. https://ifamagazine.com/study-reveals-nearly-one-in-two-are-worried-about-running-out-of-money-in-retirement/

16. Britannica. (1998, July 20). *Food.* https://www.britannica.com/topic/food

17. BTF. (n.d.). *Older patients and thyroid disease.* British Thyroid Foundation. https://www.btf-thyroid.org/older-patients-and-thyroid-disease

18. Burton-Freeman, B. M., Sandhu, A. K., & Edirisinghe, I. (2016, January 7). Red raspberries and their bioactive polyphenols: Cardiometbolic and neuronal health links. *Adv Nutr.* https://doi.org/10.3945/an.115.009639

19. Cade, J., Dunneram, y., Greenwood,D., Burley,V. (2018, April 30). *Dietary intake and age at natural menopause: results from the UK Women's Cohort Study.* https://pubmed.ncbi.nlm.nih.gov/29712719/

20. Cappuccio, F. P., Elliott, P., Pryer, J., Follman, D. A., & Cutler, J. A., (1995, November 1). Epidemiologic association between dietary calcium intake and blood pressure: A meta-analysis of published data. *Am J Epidemiol*, 142(9), 935–945. https://doi.org/10.1093/oxfordjournals.aje.a117741

21. Carey, E. (2023, July 13). *8 healthy facts about the goji berry.* https://www.healthline.com/health/goji-berry-facts

22. Central statistical release (2020, July 7). https://www.cso.ie/en/releasesandpublications/er/ilt/irishlifetablesno172015-2017/

23. Champion, C. (2021, December 22). *What you need to know about processed foods — and why it is so hard to quit them.* UCLA Health. https://www.uclahealth.org/news/article/what-you-need-to-know-about-processed-foods-and-why-it-is-so-hard-to-quit-them

24. Cibdol. (2023, August 28). *What fruit is very high in omega-3?* https://www.cibdol.com/blog/1415-what-fruit-is-very-high-in-omega-3

25. Clemente-Suárez, V. J., Beltrán-Velasco, A. I., Redondo-Flórez, L., Martin-Rodríguez, A., & Tornero-Aguilera, J. F. (2023, June 14). *Global impacts of Western diet and its effects on metabolism and health: A narrative review.* Nutrients, 15(12), 2749. https://doi.org/10.3390/nu15122749

26. Cohen, P. G. (2001, June). Aromatase, adiposity, aging and disease. The hypogonadal-metabolic-atherogenic-disease and aging condition. *Med Hypotheses*, 56(6), 702–708. https://doi.org/10.1054/mehy.2000.1169

27. Collins, J. (2023, February 2). *What top 10 triggers make perimenopause and menopause worse (and what you can do about them)*. Health & Her. https://healthandher.com/blogs/expert-advice/worsen-perimenopause-menopause-triggers

28. D'Angelo, S., Bevilacqua, G., Hammond, J., Dennison, E. M., & Walker-Bone, K. (2022, December 24). Impact of menopausal symptoms on work: Findings from women in the Health and Employment after Fifty (HEAF) study. *Int J Environ Res Public Health*, 20(1), 295. https://doi.org/10.3390/ijerph20010295

29. Davies, M. (2015, November 13). Forget Paleo — try the VICTORIAN diet! Eating onions, cabbage, beetroot and cherries meant 19th century people were healthier than we are today. *Daily Mail*. http://www.dailymail. co.ukthealth/article-3317096/Forget-Paleo-try-VICTORIAN-diet-Eating-onions-cabbage-beetroot-cherries-meant-19th-century- people-healthier-today.html

30. Dei, M. (2022, September 9). The strong Black woman. https://www.futureblackfemale.com/post/the-strong-black-woman

31. Department of Health. (2013, March 5). *Cardiovascular disease outcomes strategy: Improving outcomes for people with or at risk of cardiovascular disease*. GOV.UK. https://assets.publishing.service. gov.uk/media/5a7c0f36ed915d414762283c/9387-2900853-CVD-Outcomes_web1.pdf

32. Diamond, J. (2012, October 9). *What the doctor won't tell you about male hormone cycles*. Good Therapy https://www.goodtherapy. org/blog/male-hormonal-cycles-andropause-1009127

33. Dickenson, H. O., Nicolson, D. J., Cook, J. V., Campbell, F., Beyer, F. R., Ford, G. A., & Mason, J. (2006, April 19). Calcium supplementation for the management of primary hypertension in adults. *Cochrane Database Syst Rev*, 19(2), CD004639. https://doi.org/10.1002/14651858.cd004639.pub2

34. Dominus, S. (2023, February 1). Women have been misled about menopause. *The New York Times*. https://www.nytimes.com/2023/02/01/magazine/menopause-hot-flashes-hormone-therapy.html

35. Echeverria, V., Echeverria, F., Barreto, G. E., Echeverria, J., & Mendoza, C. (2021, May 20). Estrogenic plants: To prevent neurodegeneration and memory loss and other symptoms in women after menopause. *Front Pharmacol.*, 12, 644103. https://doi.org/10.3389/fphar.2021.644103

36. Eldred. S. M. (2023, 27 April). *Black women suffer disproportionately from menopause symptoms. Awareness could help change that.* Sahan Journal. https://sahanjournal.com/health/black-women-suffer-disproportionately-from-menopause-symptoms/

37. Encyclopaedia Britannica. (1998, July 20). *Food.* https://www.britannica. com/topic/food

38. Eneje, O. (2021, October 13). *Our crowning glory: A Black "hair" story.* Siemens. https://blog.siemens.com/2021/10/our-crowning-glory-a-black-hair-story

39. Eschner, K. (2017, February 2). The father of canning knew his process worked, but not why it worked. *Smithsonian Magazine*. https://www.smithsonianmag.com/smart-news/father-canning-knew-his-process-worked-not-why-it-worked-180961960/

40. Faubion, S. S., Enders, F., Hedges, M. S., Chaudhry, R., Kling, J. M., Shufelt, C. L., Saadedine, M., Mara, K., Griffin, J. M., & Kapoor, E. (2023). *Impact of menopause symptoms on women in the workplace.* Mayo Clinic Proceedings. https://www.mayoclinicproceedings.org/pb-assets/Health%20Advance/journals/jmcp/JMCP4097_proof.pdf

41. Gaillard, T. R. (2018, January 22). The metabolic syndrome and its components in African-American women: Emerging trends and implication. *Front Endocrinol (Lausanne)*, 8, 383. https://doi.org/10.3389/fendo.2017.00383

42. Gallicchio, L., Miller, S. R., Kiefer, J., Greene, T., Zacur, H. A., & Flaws, J. A. (2015, October). Risk factors for hot flashes among women undergoing the menopausal transition: baseline results from the Midlife Women's Health Study. *Menopause*, 22(10), 1098–1107.

43. Ganmaa, D. & Sato, A. (2005). The possible role of female sex hormones in milk from pregnant cows in the development of breast, ovarian and corpus uteri cancers. *Med Hypotheses*, 65(6), 1028–1037. https://doi.org/10.1016/j.mehy.2005.06.026

44. Gearhardt, A. N., Bueno, N. B., DiFeliceantonio, A. G., Roberto, C. A., Jiménez-Murcia, S., & Fernandez-Aranda, F. (2023, October 9). Social, clinical, and policy implications of ultra-processed food addiction. *BMJ*, 383, e075354. https://doi.org/10.1136/bmj-2023-075354

45. George, R. (2015, December 15). What science doesn't know about the menopause: What it's for and how to treat it. *The Guardian*. https://www.theguardian.com/society/2015/dec/15/what-science-doesnt-know-about-the-menopause-what-its-for-how-to-treat-it

46. Golovinskaia, O., & Wang, C. (2021, June 25). *Review of functional and pharmacological activities of berries*. Molecules, 26(13), 3904. https://doi.org/10.3390/molecules26133904

47. GOV.UK. (2017, January 20). *Policy paper Childhood obesity: A plan for action*. https://www.gov.uk/government/publications/childhood-obesity-a-plan-for-action/childhood-obesity-a-plan-for-action

48. Greek Medicine. (n.d.). *Emotions and Organs*. https://www.greekmedicine.net/hygiene/Emotions_and_Organs.html

49. Gunars, K. (2023, February 9). *10 science-backed reasons to eat more protein*. Healthline. https://www.healthline.com/nutrition/10-reasons-to-eat-more-protein

50. Gyimah, M., Azad, Z., Begun, S., Kapoor, A., Ville, L., Henderson, A., & Dey, M. (2022). *Broken ladders: The myth of meritocracy for women of colour in the workplace.* Fawcett Runnymede. https://www.fawcettsociety.org.uk/Handlers/Download.ashx?IDMF=72040c36-8cd6-4ae3-93f3-e2ad63a4b4b0

51. Harvard Health. (2013, July 1). *Eat blueberries and strawberries three times per week.* Harvard Health Publishing Harvard Medical School. https://www.health.harvard.edu/heart-health/eat-blueberries-and-strawberries-three-times-per-week

52. Herro, A. (2007, September 10). *Crop yields expand, but nutrition is left behind (Worldwatch Institute).* Desertification. https://desertification.wordpress.com/2007/09/10/crop-yields-expand-but-nutrition-is-left-behind-worldwatch-institute/

53. Horton, B., & Myers, C. (2018, June 21). *MSG: What are its potential side effects?* Eating Well. https://www.eatingwell.com/article/283965/the-msg-myth-are-there-really-side-effects

54. IMS. (2012, October 18). *Major review finds menopause does not cause weight gain, but increases belly fat.* International Menopause Society. https://www.imsociety.org/wp-content/uploads/2020/08/statement-2012-10-17.pdf

55. Irish Independent. (2015, February 23). *10 tips to balance hormones naturally.* https://www.independent.ie/life/health-wellbeing/10-tips-to-balance-hormones-naturally/31008539.html

56. James. (2023, July 21). *Cancer and food: Five herbs that could reduce risk.* The Ohio State University Comprehensive Cancer Center. https://cancer.osu.edu/blog/five-herbs-that-could-reduce-risk

57. JMU. (2017, November 9). *Good food, good mood.* James Madison University. https://www.jmu.edu/news/counselingctr/2017/01-nutrition.shtml

58. Kim, K., Wactawski-Wende, J., Michels, K. A., Plowden, T. C., Chaljub, E. N., Sjaarda, L. A., &Mumford, S. L. Dairy food intake is associated with reproductive hormones and sporadic anovulation among healthy premenopausal women. *J Nutr,* 147(2), 218–226. https://doi.org/10.3945/jn.116.241521

59. Kitsuda, Y., Wada, T., Noma, H., Osaki, M., & Hagino, H. (2021, September). Impact of high-load resistance training on bone mineral density in osteoporosis and osteopenia: A meta-analysis. *J Bone Miner Metab.,* 39(5), 787–803.

60. Knowles, L. (2012, June 24). *Doctrine of Signatures — vegetables that look like the parts they heal.* Wellness. https://balancedwellness.co.uk/doctrine-of-signatures

61. Kraft, S., (2019, May 23). Menopause and schizophrenia: A connection? Healthy Women. https://www .healthywomen.org/content/article/menopause-and-schizophrenia-connection

62. Kristy's Kitchen. (2024, August 19). *The hidden effects of MSG: Are you at risk without knowing?* https://cristyskitchenga.com/blogs/recipe-club/the-hidden-effects-of-msg-are-you-at-risk-without-knowing

63. Leeds university (2018, April 18). https://www.leeds.ac.uk/news-health/new/article/4223-The effects of diet on the start of the menopause I University of Leeds

64. Mac Bride, M. B., Rhodes, D. J., & Shuster, L. T. (2010, January). Vulvovaginal atrophy. *Mayo Clinic Proceedings*, 85(1), pp. 87–94). https://www.mayoclinicproceedings.org/article/S0025-6196(11)60314-5/fulltext

65. MacGill, M. (2017, September 4). *What is the link between love and oxytocin?* Medical News Today. https://www.medicalnewstoday.com/articles/275795.php 2017

66. MacGregor, E. A. (2009, October). Migraine headache in perimenopausal and menopausal women. *Current Pain and Headache Reports*, 13(5), 399–403. http://www.ncbi.nlm.nih.gov/pubmed/19728968

67. Macrae, F. (2011, October 2). *Male menopause affects 2m Brits but 'can be safely cured with testosterone treatment'*. Daily Mail. http://www.dailymail.co.uk/health/article02044376

68. Madhussodanian, J. (2023, June 29). Discrimination may hasten menopause in Black and Hispanic women. *Scientific American*, https://www.scientificamerican.com/article/discrimination-may-hasten-menopause-in-black-and-hispanic-women

69. Mansah-Owusu, G. (2023, April 28). It's not just hair: Hair discrimination in the workplace. *HR Magazine*. https://www.hrmagazine.co.uk/content/comment/it-s-not-just-hair-hair-discrimination-in-the-workplace/

70. Maria. (2019, November 15). *Decluttering*. Dare to Declutter. https://www.daretodeclutter.co.uk/decluttering-service/

71. Matusewicz, D. (2017, August 2). *Nine ways that processed foods are harming people.* Your Private Physician. https://yourprivatephysician. net/nine-ways-processed-foods-harming-people/

72. Mayo Clinic. (2025, February 1). *Trans fat is double trouble for heart health.* https://www.mayoclinic.org/diseases-conditions/ high-blood-cholesterol/in-depth/trans-fat/art-20046114

73. Mayo Clinic. (2024, September 20). *Arteriosclerosis/ atherosclerosis.* https://www.mayoclinic.org/diseases-conditions/ arteriosclerosis-atherosclerosis/symptoms-causes/syc-20350569

74. Mayo Clinic. (2022, May 24). *Male menopause: Myth or reality?* https://www.mayoclinic.org/healthy-lifestyle/mens-health/ in-depth/male-menopause/art-20048056

75. Metcalf, E. (2024, September 16). *Tyramine and migraines.* WebMD. https://www.webmd.com/migraines-headaches/tyramine-and-migraines

76. Meyer M.R., Clegg D.J., Prossnitz E.R., Barton M. Obesity, insulin resistance and diabetes: Sex differences and role of oestrogen receptors. Acta Physiol. 2011;203:259–26. https://pmc.ncbi.nlm. nih.gov/articles/PMC7603201/

77. Michigan News. (2022, February 23). *25 years of research shows insidious effect of racism on Black women's menopausal transition, health.* University of Michigan. https://news.umich.edu/25-years-of-research-shows-insidious-effect-of-racism-on-black-womens-menopausal-transition-health/#:~:text=Artificial%20 Intelligence,cohort%20study%20of%20midlife%20women.

78. Miller, K. (2017, April 26). *Do you really need to eat omega-3s?* Self. https://www.self.com/story/omega-3s-health-benefits

79. Miller, K., & Seegert, L. (2025, January 13). *Hypothyroidism (underactive thyroid).* WebMD. https://www.webmd.com/women/hypothyroidism-underactive-thyroid-symptoms-causes-treatments

80. Mohdin, A. (2024, September 10). Mel B among Britons taking fight against afro hair discrimination to parliament. *The Guardian.* https://www.theguardian.com/world/article/2024/sep/10/mel-b-britons-world-afro-day-hair-discrimination-parliament-equality

81. Montegnegro, X. (2004, May 1). AARP the magazine study on divorce find that women are doing the walking–but both sexes are reaping rewards in the bedroom. *AARP.* https://www.aarp.org/pri/topics/social-leisure/relationships/divorce/

82. Morrison, C. (2024, June 12). *Talking about men's health: The 'male menopause'.* Phoenix Hospital Group. https://www.phoenixhospitalgroup.com/blog/talking-about-mens-health-the-male-menopause

83. Moss, R. (2015, March 9). Women spend more than £18,000 on having periods in their lifetime, study reveals. *HuffPost.* https://www.huffingtonpost.co.uk/2015/09/03/women-spend-thousands-on-periods-tampon-tax_n_8082526.html

84. Murayama, K., Oshima, T., & Ohyama, K. (2010, February). Exposure to exogenous estrogen through intake of commercial milk produced from pregnant cows. *Paediatric International, 52*(1), 32–38. https://doi.org/10.1111/j.1442-200x.2009.02890.x

85. Murray, M. T., Pizzorno, J., & Pizzorno, L. (2005, September 20). *Encyclopaedia of Healing Foods*. Atria Books.

86. Naeem, Z. (2010, January). Vitamin D deficiency — An ignored epidemic. *Int J Health Sci (Qassim)*, 4(1), V–VI. https://pubmed.ncbi.nlm.nih.gov/21475519/

87. New Scientist. (2018, April 30). *Women who eat more pasta tend to get menopause earlier*. https://www.newscientist.com/article/2167695-women-who-eat-more-pasta-tend-to-get-menopause-earlier

88. Nguyen, P. K., Lin, S., & Heidenreich, P. (2016, January 25). A systematic comparison of sugar content in low-fat vs regular versions of food. *Nutr Diabetes*, 6(1), e193. https://doi.org/10.1038/nutd.2015.43

89. NHS. (2021, November 18). *Vitamin A: Vitamins and minerals*. National Health Service. https://www.nhs.uk/conditions/vitamins-and-minerals/vitamin-a/

90. Nienhiser, J. C. (2003, August 26). *Studies showing adverse effects of dietary soy, 1939–2014*. The Weston A. Price Foundation. https://www.westonaprice.org/health-topics/soy-alert/studies-showing-adverse-effects-of-dietary-soy-1939-2008

91. NIH. (2024, December 16). *Age-related macular degeneration (AMD)*. NIH: National Eye Institute. https://www.nei.nih.gov/learn-about-eye-health/eye-conditions-and-diseases/age-related-macular-degeneration

92. NIH. (2024a, October 28). *Atherosclerosis: Causes and Risk Factors.* National Heart, Lung, and Blood Institute. https://www.nhlbi. nih.gov/health/atherosclerosis/causes

93. NIH. (2024b, October 16). *What is menopause?* National Institute on Aging. https://www.nia.nih.gov/health/menopause/what-menopause

94. NIH. (2023, November 20). *What do we know about diet and prevention of Alzheimer's disease.* NIH: National Institute on Aging. https://www.nia.nih.gov/health/alzheimers-and-dementia/what-do-we-know-about-diet-and-prevention-alzheimers-disease

95. NIH. (2023a, April 5). *Alzheimer's disease fact sheet.* NIH: National Institute on Aging. https://www.nia.nih.gov/health/alzheimers-and-dementia/alzheimers-disease-fact-sheet

96. Northrup, C. (2012, January 3). *The wisdom of menopause: Creating physical and emotional health during the change.* Bantam.

97. Northwestern Medicine. (2024, June). *11 fun facts about your brain.* Health Beat. https://www.nm.org/healthbeat/healthy-tips/11-fun-facts-about-your-brain

98. Norton, A. (2013, September 11). *Testosterone not the whole story in 'male menopause'.* Health Day. https://www.healthday.com/health-news/women-health/testosterone-not-the-whole-story-in-male-menopause-680065.html

99. Ntuk, U., Gill, J. M. R., Mackay, D. F., Sattar, N., & Pell, J. P. (2014, June 29). Ethnic-specific obesity cutoffs for diabetes risk: cross-sectional study of 490,288 UK biobank participants. *Diabetes Care*, 37(9), 2500–2507. https://doi.org/10.2337/dc13-2966

100. Omeike, A. (2020, June 19). *Guest post: A Black woman in Scotland: A unique and complex experience. Engender.* https://www.engender.org.uk/news/blog/being-a-black-woman-in-scotland-a-unique-and-complex-experience

101. Patil, R. (2022, October 28). *Is cooking in brass and copper utensils better for health?* Let's find out! Health Shots. https://www.healthshots.com/healthy-eating/nutrition/health-benefits-of-cooking-food-in-brass-and-copper-utensils/

102. Petersen, A. (2022, April 2). Why so many women in middle age are on antidepressants. *The Wall Street Journal.* https://www.wsj.com/articles/why-so-many-middle-aged-women-are-on-antidepressants-11648906393

103. Positive Pause. (2020, April 28). *Cortisol and Menopause.* https://www.positivepause.co.uk/menopause-blog/cortisol-and-menopause

104. Rabin, R., C. (2022, June 17). Uterine cancer is on the rise, especially among Black women. *The New York Times.* https://www.nytimes.com/2022/06/17/health/uterine-cancer-black-women.html

105. Renown Health. (2018, July 5). *Early onset of puberty in girls on the rise.* https://www.renown.org/blog/early-onset-of-puberty-in-girls-on-the-rise

106. Richardson, M. K., Coslov, N., & Fugate Woods, N. (2023, April 4). Seeking health care for perimenopausal symptoms: Observations from the Women Living Better survey. *J Womens Health* (Larchmt), 32(4), 434–444. https://doi.org/10.1089/jwh.2022.0230

107. Ridley, K. (2023, June 8). *Black women denied jobs because of their hairstyles call for education. ITV News.* https://www.itv.com/news/2023-06-08/black-women-denied-jobs-because-of-their-hairstyles-call-for-education

108. Rosenbloom, C. (2017, April 18). Not all processed foods are bad for you. How they're made matters. *The Guam Daily Post.* https://www.postguam.com/entertainment/food/not-all-processed-foods-are-bad-for-you-how-theyre-made-matters/article_7bd3ed5c-231e-11e7-832e-b3cdc0ae6472.html

109. RxList. (2021, June 11). *Wild yam.* https://www.rxlist.com/supplements/wild_yam.htm

110. Schwarz, E. R., Phan, A., & Willix Jr., R. D. (2011, March). Andropause and the development of cardiovascular disease presentation — more than an epi-phenomenon. *J Geriatr Cardiol*, 8(1), 35–43. https://doi.org/10.3724/SP.J.1263.2011.00035

111. Smith, J. (2020, May 24). *How do processed foods affect your health?* Medical News Today. http://www.medicalnewstoday.com/articles/318630

112. Soley-Bori, M. (2023, March 26). *Black women face the worst health inequalities in South London.* King's College London. https://www.kcl.ac.uk/news/black-women-face-the-worst-health-inequalities-in-south-london

113. Sørensen, K.; Mouritsen, A.; Aksglaede, L.; Hagen, C.P.; Mogensen, S.S.; Juul, A (2012). Recent secular trends in pubertal timing: Implications for evaluation and diagnosis of precocious puberty. *Horm. Res. Paediatr.* https://www.mdpi.com

114. Stills, S. (2013, October 28). *How to avoid insulin resistance.* Women's Health Network. https://www.womenshealthnetwork. com/blood-sugar/how-to-avoid-insulin-resistance/

115. Sun, Y., Liu, B., Snetselaar, L. G., Robinson, J. G., Wallace, R. B., Peterson, L. L., & Bao, W. (2019, January 23). Association of fried food consumption with all cause, cardiovascular, and cancer mortality: Prospective cohort study. *BMJ*, 364. https://doi. org/10.1136/bmj.k5420

116. Tait, L. (2022, February 28). *Menopause–a self-fulfilling prophecy?* Brainz. https://www.brainzmagazine.com/post/menopause-a-self-fulfilling-prophecy

117. Tommaso, C., Verze, P., La Rocca, R., Anceschi, U., De Nunzio, C. & Mirone, V. (2017, April 21). The role of flower pollen in managing patients affected by chronic prostatitis/chronic pelvic pain syndrome: a comprehensive analysis of all published clinical trials. *BMC Urol.*, 17(1), 32. https://doi.org/10.1186/ s12894-017-0223-5

118. TUC. (2022, October). *BME women and work: TUC equality briefing.* Trade Union Congress. https://www.tuc.org.uk/sites/default/ files/2020-10/BMEwomenandwork.pdf

119. UCI. (2022, April 22). *Eating for a better night's sleep*. UCI Health. https://www.ucihealth.org/blog/2022/04/eating-for-a-better-nights-sieep

120. University of Rochester. (n.d.). *Nutrition Facts: Chrysanthemum leaves, raw, 1 cup, chopped*. University of Rochester Medical Center. https://www.urmc.rochester.edu/encyclopedia/content?contentt ypeid=76&contentid=11698-1

121. University of Washington. (n.d.). *Tips for healthy eating & healthy aging*. Healthy Aging & Physical disability: Rehabilitation Research and Training Center. https://agerrtc.washington.edu/info/factsheets/nutrition

122. UOW. (2014, April 2). *Everyday foods found to have potent anti-inflammatory properties*. University of Wollongong Australia. https://www.uow.edu.au/media/2014/everyday-foods-found-to-have-potent-anti-inflammatory-properties.php

123. Velez, A. (2021, March 10). *Menopause is different for women of color*. Health Central. https://www.healthcentral.com/condition/menopause/menopause-different-women-color

124. Ware, M. (2023, November 30). *What to know about cranberries*. Medical News Today. https://www.medicalnewstoday.com/articles/269142

125. Warner, L. (2024, July 2). *Monosodium glutamate (MSG): What it is and why you might consider avoiding foods that contain it*. Harvard Health Publishing: Harvard Medical School. https://www.health.harvard.edu/nutrition/monosodium-glutamate-msg-what-it-is-and-why-you-might-consider-avoiding-foods-that-contain-it

126. West, H. (2023, March 17). *8 foods that are high in copper.* Healthline. https://www.healthline.com/nutrition/foods-high-in-copper

127. Windhager, S., Mitteroeker, P., Rupić, I., Lauc, T., Polašek, O., & Schaefer, K. (2019, June 12). Facial aging trajectories: A common shape pattern in male and female faces is disrupted after menopause. *American Journal of Biological Anthropology*, 169(4), 678–688. https://doi.org/10.1002/ajpa.23878

128. Wurtman, J., & Frusztajer, N. T. (2009, December 22). *The serotonin power diet: Eat carbs — nature's own appetite suppressant — to stop emotional overeating and halt antidepressant-associated weight gain.* Harmony/Rodale/Convergent.

129. Xu, Q., Yan, S., Wang, C., Yu, B., Zhou, X., Luan, Q., & Na, L. (2019, May). Spicy food intake increases the risk of overweight and obesity. *Journal of Hygiene Research*, 48(3), 374–379. https://www.researchgate.net/publication/333445569_Spicy_food_

130. intake_increases_the_risk_of_overweight_and_obesity

131. Zhou, J., Huang, K., & Lei, X. G. (2013, December). Selenium and diabetes — evidence from animal studies. *Free Radic Biol Med.*, 65, 1548–1556. https://doi.org/10.1016/j.freeradbiomed.2013.07.012

An Authentic Way of being You

Conscious Dreams
PUBLISHING

Transforming diverse writers
into successful published authors

www.consciousdreamspublishing.com

authors@consciousdreamspublishing.com

Let's connect